Re

of

Radiology

Fifth Edition

Online Support at
www.indianradiology.com

- Winner of Best Clinical Website 2005 by Medgadget, Journal of Emerging Medical Technologies.

- This website has been featured in various leading International Radiology Journals.

8188867780

Review
of
Radiology

Fifth Edition

Sumer Kumar Sethi
MBBS (MAMC), MD (Radiology)
Sr. Consultant Radiologist

Director
DAMS
Delhi Academy of Medical Sciences (P) Ltd.
4-B, Pusa Road, Near Karol Bagh Metro
Station
Delhi

Director
Teleradiology Providers
Prime Teleradproviders (P) Ltd

PEEPEE
PUBLISHERS AND DISTRIBUTORS (P) LTD.

Review of Radiology

Published by
Pawaninder P. Vij
Peepee Publishers and Distributors (P) Ltd.
Head Office: 160, Shakti Vihar, Pitam Pura
New Delhi-110 034
Corporate Office: **7/31, Ansari Road, Daryaganj**
Post Box-7243, New Delhi-110002 (India)
Ph: 65195868, 23246245 9811156083
e-mail: peepee160@yahoo.co.in
e-mail: peepee160@rediffmail.com
e-mail: peepee160@gmail.com
www.peepeepub.com

© 2011 by Peepee Publishers and Distributors (P) Ltd.

First Edition: 2004
Fifth Edition: 2011

ISBN 818886778-0

Preface to the Fifth Edition

There has been a trend in the recent examinations to ask more questions of Radiology as it is very essential and upcoming subject. This book has been a very successful effort towards this cause. In this edition all recent questions from recent examinations have been added and all recent advances in the field of Radiology have been incorporated. Additional sections on mnemonics and Radiotherapy tables have been added.

With this edition, a CD has also been added in which spot cases are shown to aid recall of MCQs and to get best rank in exams. In our previous editions students had given a feedback that they want to see images as well, so in this edition we are giving complimentary CD with images and quizzes to help students grasp the subject.

Best of luck to all the readers and best of success in PG entrance.

Sumer Sethi
www.damsdelhi.com

All feedback welcome at-
director@damsdelhi.com

Preface to the First Edition

This book is mainly intended for the students appearing in the post-graduate medical admission tests of All India, different states, PGI Chandigarh, AIIMS, JIPMER, DNB, UPSC and MCI screening test for Foreign graduates etc.

Radiology is one of the subjects, which is not taught to a great detail in under graduation but forms a significant part of the postgraduate entrance examination. With the change in pattern of questions to clinical pattern especially in AIPG and AIIMS knowledge of radiological signs has become critical in reaching at the diagnosis and more importantly correct answer to the question. There is no comprehensive book available in the market for radiology, which covers all exam-oriented aspects of the subject. This book is a humble attempt to provide you with one high yield, comprehensive textbook to help you improve your performance.

This book is structured into four main sections, which are General Radiology, Systemic Radiology, Radiotherapy and a Multiple Choice Question Section. This book is written in a way that once you go through this book, you have a comprehensive idea about the subject and are able to answer majority of questions in radiology. In the first three sections various aspects of the subject have been covered with frequently asked topics or facts being marked by (*). In the last section I have given commonly asked questions to help you get the feel of the examination. In today's competitive world every subject and every question makes a difference and with limited time available to the students. It is important that you read books, which are written by experts and are worth your valuable trust.

Although, I have made my best effort to make this book a complete yet concise account of the subject. I request all my readers and critics to kindly inform me about any deficiencies. Any suggestion to improve the book will be most welcome.

Sumer K. Sethi
(Sumerdoc@yahoo.com)

Introduction

TYPES OF QUESTIONS ASKED IN RADIOLOGY MCQ

1. Radiological sign
2. Technical Question
3. Clinical problem with diagnostic radiological information

IMPORTANT

READ EVERY WORD OF THE QUESTION
Sample questions emphasizing the point

1. Young patient with sudden acute onset headache, vomiting, loss of consciousness and neck rigidity investigation of choice:
   A. X-ray
   B. MRI
   C. CT
   D. Angiography
   Answer to the question is CT scan, which is the investigation of choice in detecting acute haemorrhage.

2. Which investigation should be done in a diagnosed case of SAH?
   A. Plain X-ray
   B. CT
   C. MRI
   D. 4-vessel angiography
   Answer though the question is similarly framed answer in this question is 4-vessel angiography as now purpose is not diagnosing SAH but to look for etiology most common being aneurysm rupture.

Acknowledgements

This book is dedicated to -

To my late Grandparents for their blessings.

To my Parents Dr. Subhash Chander Sethi and Mrs. Karuna R. Sethi for being a constant source of encouragement and inspiration throughout.

To my wife Dr. Deepti Sethi nee Bahl (MS, Gynecology and Obstetrics) for her support and patience without which this project would never have been possible.

To my Brother Dr. Sidharth Kumar Sethi (MD Paediatrics) for his constant support, advice and constructive criticism and his wife Dr. Shilpa Singla (MS, Gynecology and Obstetrics, AIIMS rank 14th 2003) for her valuable help in radiotherapy part of the book.

To my Sister Sumati (M Pharm) for her guidance and advices throughout the preparation of this book.

To all my teachers especially Dr. RS Solanki (Professor, Radiodiagnosis, LHMC) and Dr MGK Murthy (Vijaya Diagnostics, Hyderabad) who always showed me the right way in life and taught me whatever I know.

To all my colleagues and seniors for their support, cooperation and suggestions in the preparation of the book.

To all friends especially Dr. Sumit Seth (MD Forensic Medicine and IFS, Columbia) and Dr. Vineet Malik (DM Cardiology), all near and dear ones and all those who helped in the preparation of the book.

To Mr. Pawaninder P. Vij, Director, Peepee Publishers and Distributors (P) Ltd., New Delhi who always used his relentless efforts to promote the book in the best possible way.

Last but not least, all my students in DAMS over the years, for inspiring and spurring me to work harder.

Contents

1. General Radiology 1
2. Systemic Radiology 24
3. Radiotherapy 98
4. Commonly Asked Questions 138
   Answers 210
5. Radiological Quiz 217
6. Some Additional Mnemonics
   in Radiology 234
7. Current Updates 242
8. Appendices 251

SPOT DIAGNOSIS IN

CD

CONCEPT OF THE BOOK

In recent few years Radiology has become a very important subject, both in clinical practice as well as undergraduate teaching. Role of physician in current day practice is not only to examine and treat the patient, but also to guide the investigations. Following the same thought process, a lot of questions are being asked in various competitive examinations about investigation of choice and important radiological signs. With a lot of technical development happening in last few years some questions are also being asked about some technical points in Radiology also.

Bearing all this in mind this book *"Review of Radiology"* is intended to be a handbook for medical students with sections on "General Radiology" which has principles and basics of various radiological procedures like Ultrasound, CT, MRI etc., "Systemic Radiology" which has all important radiological signs asked in various examinations arranged systemically, "Radiotherapy" which gives basic outline of this subject of Tumour therapy.

These sections are followed by two sections one on "Commonly Asked Questions" in various competitive examinations, with a unique way of giving the answers along with reference page numbers to the relevant topics to aid revision of important topics, other on "Image Quiz" which has images of some cases which are very commonly asked to medical students and asked as MCQs in various competitive examinations. This is again intended as a means to increase retention and aid in remembering.

A new section is added in this book on "Mnemonics" which are again some important facts which are to be remembered by students but are difficult to remember for them. So they are presented in the form of mnemonics.

A unique concept of this book is which has been largely appreciated by the students is the ONLINE SUPPORT. This comes with online support on http://www. indianradiology.com which is planned as a Radiology Magazine giving recent advances, some interesting images and an MCQ discussion and problem solving forum for the medical students. This site also features a few interesting image quizzes to help the student understand and enjoy at the same time. This site was nominated as "***Best New Medical Weblog for the Year 2004***" by echojournal.

Concluding this book is an effort to include all important points asked to a medical student in various examinations in a small handbook and also it packs along important MCQs, Images, Mnemonics and a unique Online support.

General Radiology

DISCOVERY

- X-Rays were discovered by: W.C. ROENTGEN (GERMANY)

In the latter half of the year 1895, a German scientist called Roentgen was working in his laboratory at the Physical Institute of the University of Wurzburg, Germany, experimenting with a type of discharge tube called Crooke's tube. The tube displayed a fluorescent glow when a high voltage current was passed through it. When he shielded the tube with heavy black cardboard, he found that a greenish fluorescent light could be seen on a fluorescent screen kept some 9 feet away. Roentgen concluded that a new type of ray was emitted from the tube that could pass through the black covering. The rays could pass through most substances, including the soft tissues of the body, but left the bones and most metals visible. One of his earliest photographic plates from his experiments was that of a film of his wife, Bertha's hand with a ring. Roentgen named the invisible radiations as X-rays (or unknown rays).

- Discovered on Nov 8, 1895
- Roentgen got the Nobel Prize in–1901*

PROPERTIES

- Wave length—0.1-1 A°*
- X-ray are ElectroMagnetic Radiation*
- Wave particle theory—can behave both as wave and particle.
- Radiation passes through the patient –USEFUL BEAM AND SCATTER RADIATION
- SPEED OF X-rays is 3×10^8 m/sec= that of light**
- Has photographic effect.

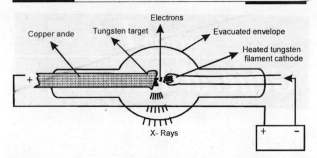

Figure. 1.1

HOW ARE X-RAYS PRODUCED?

An X-ray tube has a cathode and an anode, cathode is a tungsten filament which produces electrons when heated (**PROCESS IS** THERMOIONIC EMISSION); anode or the target is made of Tungsten.

X-RAYS ARE PRODUCED WHEN ELECTRON BEAM PRODUCED FROM CATHODE (TUNGSTEN FILAMENT) STRIKES THE ANODE.

ANODE can be either stationary or rotating with rotating anode having BETTER HEAT DISSIPIATION

Please note: target is not of tungsten in Mammography-it's made of Molybdenum

X-RAY FILM

Emulsion: Photo sensitive Material–Silver halide
PRINCIPLE OF IMAGE FORMATION-Photoelectric effect once the image is exposed, it has to be developed and fixed.

- Development–hydroquinone + metol/ phenindione
- Fixer- hypo- Na thiosulphate.

SPECIAL X-RAYS TUBES

- Mammography:
  - High contrast desirable.
    Conventional X-ray tube has glass window and aluminium filter.
  While the mammography has:
  - Molybdenum target
  - Molybdenum filter
  - Beryllium window

EXPOSURE FACTORS

- Exposure factors are:
  1. kVP- determines the beam Penetration* (kilovolt peak)
  2. mAS- determines the amount of film Blackening* (milliampere second)
- Contrast: Is mainly influenced by KVP* (remembering TIP- K for Kontrast) low KVP implies High contrast and vice-versa
- Obese Patient REQUIRES A HIGH KVP as they require more penetration.

FILM-FOCUS DISTANCE FOR ROUTINE RADIO-GRAPHY IS 100 cm WHILE FOR CXR IS 180 cm or 6 ft TO REDUCE MAGNIFICATION.*

FEW TECHNICAL POINTS

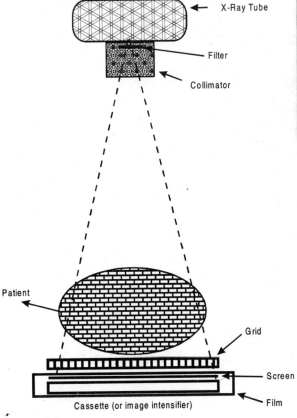

Figure. 1.2

Intensifying Screen

- Principle- PHOSPHORENCE
- MATERIAL-Calcium tungstate
  New technology: Rare earth phosphors screens
(Principle-X-rays are converted to light photons as films
are more sensitive to light than X-rays and one X-ray photon produces around 50 light photons, so less X-ray exposure is required with intensifying screens)

Filter

Aluminium or aluminium copper combination absorbs low
energy X-rays–decrease patient exposure*

Grid

Has multiple parallel lead lines with intervening radiolucent
material which absorb the scatter radiation and improves
contrast*

Collimators and Cones

Restrict field size*
Also decreases scatter radiation.

Safe Light

This is the light used in dark room in radiology, which does
not affect the radiographs. Commonly used is RED and
with 15 Watt illumination.

CONVENTIONAL TECHNIQUES

Fluoroscopy

Real time X-Ray Imaging*
Phosphor used
Conventional fluoroscopy– material used is Ag activated
ZnCdS (silver activated zinc cadmium sulfide)
Image Intensifier –Cesium Iodide

Tomography

Only one section of body is kept in sharp focus rest all is
blurred.

Xeroradiography

- Uses Selenium as image receptor*
- Electrostatic Latent image
- Advantage: High Edge enhancement*
- Disadvantage: High radiation exposure*
- Used in breast imaging.

COMPUTED TOMOGRAPHY

Discovered by-Godfrey Hounsfield
In 1972, by EMI limited (Electro musical instrument)*, Middlesex England
He received the Nobel Prize in 1979*
Basic Principle: Thin section of body are achieved to create axial sections of the body.

Advances CT Technology

- **Spiral CT**: Uses the principle of **Volumetric Acquisition** with simultaneous patient motion and image acquisition. No respiratory misregistration.
- **Multislice CT**: Latest innovation in CT technology Cardiac applications* (especially coronary CT angiography and coronary calcium estimation). Advantage: High resolution / high speed
- **Electron beam CT:** Fast scanner useful for cardiac applications inferior to multislice CT
- **High resolution CT:**
  Investigation of choice in
- ILD (Intestinal lung disease)
- Bronchiectasis.

Principle of HRCT

- Thin collimation
- High resolution BONE algorithm for image reconstruction.
- Small field of view

CECT: Usually used for all cranial applications; Usually uses Iodinated Contrast

NCCT indicated for: (Non-contrast CT)

- Head injury/stroke
- Acute hemorrhage
- SAH

Haemorrhage on CT

- ACUTE SAH < 48 hrs – **CT investigation of choice**
- Chronic SAH > 48 hrs – **MRI investigation of choice**
  *Biconvex hyperdense – extradural hemorrhage – (Fig. 1.3A) Arterial
  *Concavo-convex – Subdural hemorrhage – Venous (Fig. 1.3B). Density of hemorrhage decreases with time and gradually approaches that of CSF.

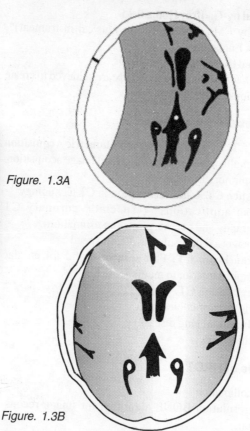

Figure. 1.3A

Figure. 1.3B

CT Density SCALE- hounsfield units (**HU**)* Water 0HU*, -1000HU: Air*, Calcification +1000HU*, Fat -100HU*, Hemorrhage 60-70HU*

3D **Reconstruction possible with spiral and multislice CT** especially useful for craniovertebral anomalies, acetabular injury and spinal bony injury etc.

CT ANGIOGRAPHY-**USES** MIP (**maximum intensity projection**) and SSD (**surface shaded display**)

CALCIFICATION best detected on CT **
CT is best for Pancreatic imaging.

USG (ULTRASONOGRAPHY)

- 3-5 MHz- Routine Abdominal Imaging*
- Crystal: PZT Lead Zirconate Titanate*
- Principle: Piezo-electric effect**
- Speed in sound in body 1540 m/s
- For superficial USG – 7-10 MHz ** (use higher frequency for superficial parts)
- Best for solid vs. cystic lesions, minimal fluid etc.

Modes in USG

- A mode–AMPLITUDE MODE
  a. Ophthalmology
  b. Orbital biometry**
- B mode/ GRAY SCALE—For all routine applications
- M-mode – Echo cardiography*.

Advantages
No radiation** / portable

Disadvantage
Operator dependance
Delerious effect on small organism of USG is by **Acoustic cavitation.**
Note—Following investigations do not use ionizing radiation:
  a. Ultrasonography.
  b. Thermography.
  c. MRI.

DOPPLER

Principle: described by Christian Johann Dopple-Frequency shift of moving object recorded
- Pulsed Doppler-gives the exact velocity waveform
- **Colour doppler**–Direction Information–**blue** away from the transducer, **red** is towards the transducer**
- Power doppler–Slow Flow detection. Like tumoral vascularity.

Common indications of doppler include PVD, Carotid atherosclerosis, Portal HT, IUGR, PIH, RenoVascular HT etc.

SECTION ONE

MRI (MAGNETIC RESONANCE IMAGING)

Principle–same as NMR, which is an analytical tool in chemistry

PROTON (H^+) **Acts as Dipole with Magnetic Dipole Movement and Gyromagnetic Property.** **

Constant Magnetic field—addition of RF pulse—moves the dipole and then the RF pulse is switched off-then when the proton returns to the previous state the signal known as FID (Free Induction Decay) is generated. *

Nobel prize for medicine 2003-Laterbuer and Mansfield for MRI **.

Magnetic Field

Generated by three geometries:

* **Permanent magnets** –0.1-0.3 T
* **Resistive air core**
* **Super conducting** 2-4 T

  T_1 – spin lattice relaxation time **

  T_2- Spin-Spin relaxation time **

  (How to remember Spin—Spin Implies Spin-2 so T2)

Magnets, Wires and Liquid Coolants (important source of Qs in last few exams). An MR scanner has a large electromagnet around a human-sized tube where the patient or test subject lies. The larger the number of windings, the greater the magnetic field. Magnetic field strength is measured in Tesla (T). **Clinical imaging scanners have magnets with field strengths ranging from .02 to 1.5T*** average one Tesla.**

To maintain a state of super-conductivity, the magnet is kept under conditions of intense cold. Its coiled wires rest inside a double-walled apparatus that is bathed in **liquid helium**, which is only 4.2 degrees Celsius above absolute zero, the point at which molecules stop moving. The apparatus is kept in a vacuum and left inside a tank filled with **liquid nitrogen**. **

Superconductors offer no resistance to electricity. This means that once an electric current is introduced into the coils, the current will continue at full strength for years without the need of more electrical input.

The entire MR scanner installation is enclosed in a stainless steel or copper shield known as a **Faraday cage** *** that blocks out radio frequency signals from local radio and TV stations that might influence the MR signals.

Magnetic devices called gradient coils play an important role in scanning. **Gradient coils** are used to vary the strength of the main magnetic field. Although the coils are securely anchored to the frame of the scanner, the immense magnetic forces that come into play during scanning cause the coils to bang against their mooring. This banging is the loud rhythmic noise that is associated with MR scanning.

Important, too, are **radio frequency coils** that transmit and receive radio frequency signals.

OTHER APPLICATIONS OF FARADAY CAGE

- Electromyography (EMG).
- Evoked potential recordings (EVP).
- Electroencephalograms (EEG).

MR Signal Characteristics

- CSF: hypointense on T1 WI, hyperintense on T2WI**
- **Grey/White Matter:** Grey matter is grey and white matter is white on T1WI and relationship is reversed on T2WI**
- Most tumors are hyperintense on T2WI except **Melanoma**-hyperintense on T1 WI & hypointense on T2WI**
- **FAT**—hyperintense on T1 WI, less hyperintense on T2WI**
- **Flowing blood**-Signal void**.

How to Remember

"WW 2" (World War II):
- **W**ater is **W**hite in a T**2** scan.
- Conversely, a T1 scan shows fat as being whiter.

Signal Void on MRI

- Flow in vessels
- Air/gas
- Scar
- Hemosiderin
- Calcification
- Metallic foreign body.

MRA (Magnetic Resonance Angiography)

Time of flight and Phase contrast sequences used; usually no contrast is used

Important Points

Contrast USED IN MRI—Gadolinium DTPA (V. IMPORTANT)**

No contrast used in MRCP, MR myelography etc. they use Heavily T2 weighted **sequences**

Ischaemic Stroke detected earlier on MRI (esp. DW MRI) diffusion weighted imaging. **

   Hemorrhage detected earlier on NCCT head. **

   MRI is best modality for posterior fossa lesions.

Drawbacks of MRI

- Cortical bone
- Acute hemorrhage
- Calcium

CT better modality for these conditions**

- Metallic foreign body
- Claustrophobia**
- When suspecting a **metallic Foreign body in Eye** MRI is contraindicated; also with **pacemakers** and **cochlear implants** because they experience a torque in the magnetic field**.

Advantages of MRI

- High soft tissue contrast
- No ionizing radiation **(Safe in Pregnancy)**
- **Multiplanar** imaging
- Better for bone marrow
- All spinal imaging – MRI, posterior-fossa—MRI.
- **Doesn't use iodinated contrast** so safe in iodine allergy.

RULES IN RADIOLOGY

A. Bone metastatis—Bone scan is the preferred investigation **

   Except – Spine—MRI even better than bone scan. **

B. For Lung imaging—CT is usually the preferred modality *Except**

- Pancoast tumor or superior sulcus tumour (as it involves branchial plexus and sympathetic chain)

- Posterior Mediastinal masses
  In these conditions MRI is better than CT
C. For all brain tumours best investigation is Contrast enhanced MRI.

IODINATED CONTRAST MEDIA

a. **Ionic High Osmolar****–Urograffin–Ditrazoate sodium and meglumine salts
   - Conray (lothalamate)
b. Non ionic: **Low Osmolar****
   Ioversol (optiray) MONOMER
   Iohexol (omnipaque) MONOMER
   Iodixanol DIMER.

Low Osmolar Agents are Safer

Contrast Reaction: Idiosyncratic—**Anaphylactoid reaction not true anaphylaxis**** (as there is no true antigen—Antibody reaction.
Non-Idiosyncratic dose dependent.
Treatment for acute bronchospasm is **s/c adrenaline.**

Iodinated Contrast

Radio-opacity is dependent on the **iodine concentration** of the solution and is therefore dependent on the *number of iodine atoms per molecule* and the *concentration of the molecules in the solution.*

   Iodine: particle ratio—The ratio of the *number of iodine atoms per molecule* to the *number of osmotically active particles per molecule of solute* in solution is a fundamental criterion. This iodine: particle ratio for current products varies from 3:2 for conventional high-osmolar ionic monomers (HOCM) to 6:1 for nonionic dimmers.

   The adverse reactions caused by hyperosmolality of the contrast medium include:
   a. *Erythrocyte damage.*
   b. *Endothelial damage.*
   c. *Blood–brain barrier damage.*
   d. *Hypervolaemia.*
   e. Cardiac depression.

   <u>Adrenaline (epinephrine), 0.3–1.0 ml, 1/1000 solution (children 0.01 ml kg^{-1} body weight) by deep subcutaneous or intramuscular injection repeated at 10–20 min intervals, provides the most rapid and reliable relief for</u>

bronchospasm, angioneurotic oedema, and other anaphylactoid symptoms.

Contrast Induced Nephropathy

Patients with pre-existing renal disease, particularly those with the renal complications of diabetes mellitus, have an increased risk of an adverse reaction which may precipitate renal failure

Tests of renal function after contrast medium-serum creatinine and urea levels and the GFR are crude measurements of renal function and nephrotoxicity. More sophisticated and sensitive methods include the detection in the blood and urine of enzymes, e.g. N-acetyl-β-D-glucosaminidase (NAG), alanine aminopeptidase (AAP), and α-glutamyl transpeptidase (αGT). Immuno-enzymatic techniques with monoclonal antibodies promise to become more effective methods of assessing the renal damage caused by contrast media, but enzymuria is probably not a good marker for RCM-induced nephrotoxicity.

PROCEDURES

GIT Imaging

In gastrointestinal tract we usually use barium as contrast agent

Where Not to use Barium sulphate:
- Tracheo esophageal fistula- use Dianosil—water soluble non-ionic agent***
- Perforation peritonitis–use Gastograffin-Ionic water soluble agent**

Procedures: Single contrast uses barium alone

Double contrast: uses **air and barium** – better for small mucosal lesion **

Ba swallow uses barium paste (for esophagus)

Ba meal 95%w/v BaSO$_4$ (for stomach and duodenum)

Ba meal follow through 50% (for small bowel)

Ba enema 25% (for large bowel)

Investigation of choice for small bowel—Enteroclysis or small bowel enema**

Bowel thickening on USG gives rise to **Pseudokidney Appearance**.

BILIARY IMAGING

OCG

- Oral cholecystography
- Dye used
  Iopaonic acid (telepaque)**
  Calcium ipodate (bilioptin)
- Also called **Graham – Cole** test*
- Most gall bladder pathologies – USG is the investigation of choice*
  Except: **Acute cholecytitis—TC^{99} HIDA scan** is the investigation of choice**.

IV Cholangiography

Uses Biligraffin but it is a toxic dye so not a popular procedure.

JAUNDICE

ERCP (endoscopic retrograde cholangiopancreato-graphy): low site of jaundice like CBD obstruction it can be combined with papillotomy and stone removal*
PTC (percutaneous transhepatic cholangiography): High site of jaundice like klatskin tumour.
USG for initial evaluation of surgical jaundice**.
Radionuclide scanning is also done for evaluation of biliary atresia but the gold standard is Peroperative chol-angiography.

MRCP (magnetic resonance cholangiopancreatography)

- No contrast material used; **heavily T2WI used.**
- No endoscopy.
- CAN BE DONE Post Whipples, gastrojejunostomy.

IVP (INTRAVENOUS PYELOGRAPHY)

**Nephrogram—contrast is in PCT (proximal convoluted tubules) **
- Pyelogram—Collecting system / Pelvis
- Dose of contrast is-300 mg / kg; in renal failure—600 mg / I_2 or double dose for contrast
- Films taken at- 1,5,10,15 min.
- Upper ureters – Supine film better

- Lower ureters—Prone film better
- IVP should be carefully performed in diabetics, multiple myeloma and dehydration should be avoided in these cases (relative contraindication).

Urethrography: Anterior urethra is best visualized by retrograde urethrography and posterior urethra is best seen by micturating (voiding) cystourethrography. Reflux is best seen on MCU.

UPPER TRACT URODYNAMIC STUDY OR WHITAKER TEST

Kidney is perfused at a rate 10 ml/min with a nephrostomy catheter and pelvicalyceal pressure and bladder pressure are measured; if the differential pressure between kidney and bladder is >22 cm water it implies ureteric obstruction, <15cm water is normal.

ANGIOGRAPHY

Non-ionic agent performed.

Technique

Earlier used—Direct puncture

Now use catheter technique—via **femoral puncture****
Technique SELDINGER technique**

DSA or digital subtraction angiography used as low volume contrast is required for diagnostic quality images.

Uses Digital subtraction to obtain a bone free image.

Carotid angiography: first done by MONIZ.

Conventional 4-vessel angiography done by injecting in 2 internal carotids and 1 vertebral. Fourth vessel fills by reflux**

Renal hypertension–Screening–captopril DTPA scanning (MR angiography has best sensitivity and specificity among non-invasive modalities)

Gold std. – Angiography.

MISCELLANEOUS

Myelography–use only non-ionic contrast media IONIC IS NEVER USED**

(CT: Myelography) can be done as an add on conventional CT

Myodil (Phenydylate) OILY contrast media** –earlier used for myelography caused a high incidence of arachnoiditis so not used nowadays. **

For renovascular hypertension screening use Captopril DTPA scanning, gold standard-renal angiography.

Cardiac Imaging

Perfusion Scanning
Thallium 201(half life 73 hr)—infarct– Cold spot on thallium scanning**
Reversible ischaemia will be cold on exercise and normal on rest while irreversible infarct will be cold on both. So thallium determines the reversibility of a lesion. **
Tc^{99} **pyrophosphate**-infarct binding agent – hot spot on scanning*** (infarct scintigraphy).

Functional Isotope Imaging in Heart

To evaluate ventricular function can be done by two methods first pass method and gated equilibrium studies, gated studies are also known as multiple gated acquisition (MUGA).

Ventricular Function Assessment

<u>**Techniques using three-dimensional MRI image acquisition are the most accurate methods for determining cardiac dimensions and mass.**</u> Ventricular volumes can be more rapidly estimated, with reasonable accuracy, using two-dimensional images acquired from US, CT, and MRI and applying one of a variety of formulae (such as Simpson's rule). These formulae make assumptions about ventricular geometry (the normal left ventricle is assumed to be a prolate ellipse) and calculate approximate ventricular volumes from two-dimensional dimensions. These methods become less accurate in the dilated ventricle.

Lungs

For pulmonary embolism ventilation-perfusion scanning or V/Q scanning.

Ventilation Agents:
- Xe 133 t1/2 5.7 days
- Kr 81- t1/2 13 sec
- Technegas. Tc99 labelled aerosols

Perfusion Agent
- Tc^{99} MAA macro aggregates of albumin

Highly Suggestive Finding

V/Q MISMATCH implies a pulmonary infarct. Pulmonary infarct shows normal ventilation and abnormal perfusion. A matched defect is less likely to be an infarct as normal pulmonary vessel constricts in response to hypoxia giving rise to a matched defect as opposed to a mismatch in infarction.

Thyroid

I^{131} t1/2-8days*. Dose-50-100 μCi.

Used for localising and treating metastatis after thyroid ablation**

I^{123} t1/2-13 hours used for thyroid functional evaluation. Dose-100-300 μCi. Tc^{99}—2-10 μCi.

Like iodine, radioiodine is taken up and concentrated in thyroid follicular cells because they have a membrane sodium-iodide transporter. Compared with normal thyroid follicular cells, thyroid cancer cells have reduced expression of the transporter, which may account for the low 131-I uptake in thyroid cancer tissue. <u>**131-I causes acute thyroid-cell death by emission of short path-length (1 to 2 mm) beta rays. The uptake of 131-I by thyroid tissue can be visualized by scanning to detect the gamma radiation that is also emitted by the isotope.**</u>

GI Bleeding

TC^{99} RBC can detect as much as 0.1 ml/min of bleeding as opposed to 0.5 ml/min by angiography.***

GASTROINTESTINAL BLEEDING

A radionuclide ^{99m}Tc-tagged erythrocyte scan during the acute bleeding may be helpful in identifying the area of origin of the bleeding. Although it is advocated as capable of detecting blood loss as slow as 0.1 to 0.2 mL/min, a loss of 0.5 mL/min is more realistic; the scan can be repeated for up to 30 h when bleeding is intermittent Arteriography will identify a bleeding site when the bleeding rate is higher, e.g., 1 to 2 mL/min. Arteriography also may identify a tumor blush or an arteriovenous malformation or angiodysplasia. Tagged-erythrocyte scans and arteriographic investigations may demonstrate a small-intestinal source and may localize it to the upper or lower small intestine. If the specific arterial arcade affected can be identified on angiography, it is helpful to select the specific branch and leave the catheter in place for intra-operative localization. At operation, it may be necessary to transilluminate the small bowel or to carry out intraoperative enteroscopy, which is an effective tool in selected patients with occult gastrointestinal bleeding and correctly identifies a treatable source and prevents rebleeding in 41 percent of patients.

GI bleeding: *TC^{99} RBC can detect as much as 0.1 ml/ min of bleeding as opposed to 0.5 ml/min by angiography.*

Bone Scanning

Phosphonates the preferred compound (Subramaniam *et al*)

Commonly used MDP TC^{99} methylene diphosphonate **

3 phases: Perfusion phase (immediate), blood pool phase (5-10 min) and delayed or bone uptake (2-3 hrs) phase.

Acute Osteomyelitis Vs Cellulitis acute osteomyelitis is hot on all three phases cellulitis only on first two phases. Radionuclide bone scanning is best for early detection of osteomyelitis.

Also used to detect skeletal metastasis.

Parathyroid Imaging

Thallium - Tc^{99} subtraction scanning**.

Nowadays Sestamibi scanning is used for parathyroid imaging.

Reticuloendothelial System

Tc^{99} sulfur colloid scanning**

Kupffer cells in liver take up Tc^{99} sulfur colloid scanning** (also FNH which is a Kupffer cell rich tumour).

Hepatic Scintigraphy

Hepatic scintigraphy or the liver scan, as it is commonly referred to involves intravenous injection of a radioactive isotope tagged to a colloid which is predominantly taken up selectively by the Kupffer cells of the liver. A small percentage is also trapped by the reticuloendothelial system of the spleen and bone marrow.

The scintigraphic features of focal lesions depend on the presence or absence of Kupffer cells. In space occupying lesions such as cysts, abcesses, primary and secondary neoplasms there are no Kupffer cells and they appear as cold spots. In focal nodular hyperplasia (FNH), there is a predominance of Kupffer cells in more than 50 per cent of cases and the lesion is exhibited as a hot nodule. It is also a highly vascular tumour and irrespective of the number of Kupffer cells can be seen as an area of increased activity in the perfusion phase (initial blood flow phase). Hepatic adenoma is devoid of Kupffer cells and is depicted as a cold area on liver scan in 80 per cent of cases.

Ectopic Gastric Mucosa

TC^{99} pertechnnate–e.g. in MECKEL's diverticulum.

MIBG Scanning Useful in

- Phaeochromocytoma
- Neuroblastoma
- Ganglioneuroma
- Paraganglioma.

PET

Positron emission tomography.
It is a Functional Imaging method.
Agent: 18 Fluorodeoxy glucose (18 FDG) for **metabolic agent,** localizes tumour because of its uptake in glycolysis.
Perfusion agents: Labelled NH_3, Rb-81.

PET studies with FDG have been used to locate cerebral tumors, distinguish high grade tumors from low grade and benign tumors, and in post treatment to distinguish recurrence from radiation necrosis.

Also useful in evaluation of epileptic foci, dementia etc.

Half life of F-18 is 110 minutes.

SPECT (SINGLE PHOTON EMISSION COMPUTED TOMOGRAPHY)

Uses Tc^{99} labelled agents only so easily available as compared to PET which use cyclotron produced agents. Gives a three dimensional image as opposed to a planar image by routine radionuclide imaging.

RADIATION PROTECTION

Ionizing radiation—$H_2O \rightarrow H^+$ & OH^-, leads to Free Radicle induced DNA damage.

Effects of Radiation

a. Stochastic effects – which are not dose dependent, they have no threshold for their occurrence, like genetic effects, mutations, carcinogenesis etc.
b. Non stochastic–dependent on the radiation dose or they have a threshold for their occurrence.
c. The cell cycle for mammalian cells can be divided into four phases: mitosis (M), followed by G1, followed by the DNA synthetic phase (S), then G2, and into mitosis again.
   • In general, cells are most radiosensitive in late M and G2 phases and most resistant in late S. **
   • The pattern of resistance and sensitivity correlates with the level of sulfhydryl compounds in the cell. Sulfhydryls are natural radio protectors and tend to be at their highest levels in S and at their lowest near mitosis. **
   • The presence or absence of molecular oxygen dramatically influences the biological effect of X-rays.
   • The oxygen enhancement ratio (OER) is the ratio of doses without and with oxygen to produce the same biological effect. **
   • Radiation therapy is the use of X-rays, gamma rays, electrons, etc. to treat rapidly dividing malignant and non-malignant tumors. Intraoperative radiotherapy uses electrons to produce ionizations in cancer cells. Its attraction lies in the direct irradiation of the surgically exposed tumor. Intraoperative radiotherapy (IORT) is a specialised treatment technique that uses either electron or orthovoltage irradiation at the time of surgery directly to tumour or tumour bed. *

Basic principle of radiation protection is—ALARA—as low as reasonably achievable.

LATEST ICRP (International council for radiation protection) Recommendations—
Maximum Permissible dose for various groups is:
• Occupation Exposure—20 msv per annum (averaged over a period of five years).

* General public – 1 msv per annum
* Pregnancy –2 msv for the duration of the declared term.

Other Relevant Facts

* One CXR is equivalent to 0.06 msv and factors for it are 60 kVp and 16 mAs
* Lead apron recommended thickness– 0.5 mm **.

RADIATION UNITS

1. **Roentgen**–unit of radiation exposure SI unit is coloumb/kg*
2. Unit of Absorbed radiation – **RAD** *
   SI unit GRAY
   1 **Gray** = 100 RAD
3. Unit of Biological effectiveness or equivalent dose – **REM****
   SI unit-Sievert
   1 sv = 100 REM
4. Radioactivity
   1 **Becquerel**=1 disintegration/sec
   1 **Curie** = 3.7×10^{10} disintegrations/sec**.

RADIATION MONITORING

Commonly used technique—**TLD** or thermo luminiscent dosimetry.**

BEST VIEW

* Pneumothorax—PA (expiration)
* Trauma—skull lateral (cross table horizontal beam)
* Pituitary—coned down lateral view
* Orbit—Caldwell view (PA 20 degree caudal)
* Recurrent shoulder dislocation—Strykers view
* Optic canal—Rhees view
* Cervical intervertebral foramen—oblique view
* Sacroiliac joints, parsinterarticularis—oblique view
* Left atrial enlargement—Barium swallow (Right anterior oblique)
* Left lung—right anterior oblique
* Right lung—left anterior oblique
* Minimal pleural effusion—lateral decubitus
* Fracture scaphoid—oblique
* Petrous bone—townes/stenvers view
* Patellofemoral articulation—skyline view
* Maxillary sinus, PNS—waters/occipitomental view
* Middle lobe lesion/interlobar fissure effusion—lordotic view.

Effective doses for common radiological examinations expressed in terms of the equivalent number of chest X-rays and length of exposure to background radiation that would give the same dose

Examination	Typical effective dose (mSv)	Equivalent no. of chest X-rays	Equivalent length of background exposure
X-ray examinations			
Limbs and joints (except hip)	<0.01	<0.5	<1.5 days
Chest (single PA radiograph)	0.02	1	3 days
Skull	0.07	3.5	11 days
Thoracic spine	0.7	35	4 months
Lumbar spine	1.3	65	7 months
Hip	0.3	15	7 weeks
Pelvis	0.7	35	4 months
Abdomen	1.0	50	6 months
IVU	2.5	125	14 months
Barium swallow	1.5	75	8 months
Barium meal	3	150	16 months
Barium follow-through	3	150	16 months
Barium enema	73.5	350	3.2 years
CT head	2.3	115	1 year
CT chest	8	400	3.6 years
CT abdomen or pelvis	10	500	4.5 years
Radionuclide studies			
Lung Ventilation (Xe-133)	0.3	15	7 weeks
Lung perfusion (Tc-99m)	1	50	6 months
Kidney (Tc-99m)	1	50	6 months
Thyroid (Tc-99m)	1	50	6 months
Bone (Tc-99m)	4	200	1.8 years
Dynamic Cardiac (Tc-99m)	6	300	2.7 years
PET head (F-18 FDG)	5	250	2.3 years

CHEST IMAGING

RESPIRATORY SYSTEM

IMAGING MODALITIES

a. CXR for all X-rays film focus distance is 100 cm while for **CXR its 180 cm or 6 feet** to reduce magnification, normal chest X-ray is done in full inspiration, erect facing the film.
b. CT
c. MRI
d. HRCT
e. Ventilation perfusion scanning

<u>**PA View versus AP View Chest**</u> (posteroanterior and anteroposterior)

Chest in AP view scapulae overlie the upper lungs, clavicles project over the apices disk spaces of lower cervical spine are more clearly seen in PA view neural arches are visualized.

PLEURA

Pleural Lesions

a. Pleural effusion MINIMAL AMOUNT REQUIRED TO BE DETECTED:
   LATERAL VIEW-75 ml pleural fluid*
   PA VIEW-100-200 ml pleural fluid*
   Lateral decubitus-<10 ml pleural fluid **
b. **Vanishing or pseudo tumor**: loculated effusion in interlobar fissure—seen in CHF***
   Lordotic View** best for:
   ➢ Middle lobe pathologies
   ➢ Inter lobar effusion.
c. **Lateral decubitus view of the same side:** best view to detect minimal effusion***
d. USG best investigation to detect minimal fluid.

Pneumothorax

a. Expiratory film is the best projection for detection of pneumothorax
b. CT better
c. No role for USG in pneumothorax as air causes reverbration artifacts on USG.

Pneumomediastanium

- **Spinnaker sail sign**: air outlining sail shaped thymus
- **Continuous diaphragm sign**: (air collects beneath the pericardium so the central part of diaphragm becomes visible).

Pneumopericardium

Gas does not extend beyond aortic knuckle and changes with change in position.

Pleural Calcification

Causes**

a. **Asbestosis:** involves parietal pleura, Diaphragmatic pleura calcification classical for Asbestosis.
b. **Empyema and old hemothorax** also cause pleural calcification however they involve the visceral pleura and usually unilateral
   - Best method to demonstrate pleural plaque is HRCT.

Pleural Malignancy

Primary—Mesothelioma**
Secondary
1. Thymoma *
2. Bronchogenic Ca
3. Breast.

NORMAL CHEST

Best View

For Right lung is Left Anterior Oblique and for Left Lung Right Anterior Oblique. **

Radiological Hilum***

- FORMED BY-Upper lobe veins, Pulmonary artery, bronchus***

SECTION TWO

- Pulmonary Artery forms the major part of the radiological hilar shadow**
- Lower lobe veins don't form a part of the radiological hilum**
- Left hilum is 2.5 cm higher than the right as left pulmonary artery passes above the bronchus and right passes anterior to its bronchus**.

Thymus

- **Sail Sign** thymus has a characteristic triangular shape
- **Wave Sign of Muvley** indentations on soft thymus due to ribs
- **Notch Sign.**

Few Important Radiological Facts

Left dome of diaphragm is lower than the right because heart pushes the left dome down (Imp MCQ).

Left hilum is higher than right hilum (left pulmonary artery is superior to bronchus and right pulmonary artery is anterior).

Pleural lesion forms an obtuse angle with the chest wall; while parenchymal lesion forms an acute angle.

Solitary pulmonary nodule-lesion less than 6 cm in size and >6 cm is mass.

Calcification common in benign lesion: Eccentric calcification can be seen in malignant lesion**.

Silhouette Sign

Given by Felson: Permits localization of a lesion on a film by studying the diaphragm and mediastinal outlines.
1. Middle lobe and lingular lobe pathology will obliterate the corresponding cardiac border**.
2. Anterior versus Posterior mediastinal lesion anteriorly placed lesion will silhoutte the cardiac border while posterior lesion will not.

PULMONARY INFECTIONS

Radiology of Pulmonary Tuberculosis:***

Primary TB:
- Ghon's lesion: Subpleural consolidation + lymphatic + enlarged lymph nodes.

- Lymphadenopathy is characteristic of primary infection (also in Tuberculosis with AIDS).
- Consolidation can occur anywhere in the lung (More common subpleural sites in lower lobe).

Secondary TB:

- Cavitation
- Fibrosis
- Involves Apical segments of upper and lower lobes
- V. UN COMMON IN ANTERIOR SEGMENT OF UPPER LOBE**.

Hematogenous spread of TB leads to miliary shadowing
Endobronchial spread: Tree in bud appearance**.

Rasmussen aneurysm: Pulmonary artery in cavity TB may cause hemoptysis**

—In hemoptysis—First vessel to be studied-Bronchial artery. Lymphnode show peripheral enhancement on CT because of necrosis.

Pneumonia

Pneumococcal—more commonly basal, klebsiella more common right upper lobe, bulging fissure, mycoplasma earliest CXR change is fine reticulo-nodular shadows followed by consolidation. Viral pneumonias may show-peribronchial shadowing, reticulonodular shadows and consolidation.

Bulging Fissure

- **Klebsiella** pneumonia (Freidlander's bacillus)
- Lung abscess
- Ca bronchus

Hydatid Lung

- No or rare calcification in lung.
- 'Water lily' sign OR CAMALOTE SIGN**

Hydatid cyst forms three layers:

Pericyst due to fibrous host reaction, ectocyst and the endocyst containing brood capsules.

Aspergillosis in Lung

1. **Aspergilloma**
   CXR show density surrounded by air in the cavity (air crescent sign).

AIR CRESCENT SIGN

- **Aspergilloma or fungal ball**
- Inspissated pus in a cavity
- Tumour or clot within the cavity
- Hydatid cyst.

---

2. **Invasive aspergillosis**
   In immunocompromised persons
   CT Halo appearance due to surrounding haemorrhagic inflammation.
3. **Allergic bronchopulmonary aspergillosis** type III immune reaction, central bronchiectasis, 'gloved finger appearance'

Pneumocystitis Carnii

CXR normal in 10% may show perihilar and mid/lower zone ground glass infiltrates, lymphadenopathy pleural effusion less common. Pneumothorax is well recognized complication.

Bronchiectasis

Morphological Types (increasing severity)
1. Cylindrical
2. Varicose
3. Cystic

Radiological Signs**

- 'Signet-ring' sign—bronchus is larger than the accompanying vessel.
- Tram track sign—Lack of peripheral tapering (cylindrical bronchiectasis).
- String of beads appearance alternate dilatation and constriction (varicoid bronchiectasis).
- Cluster of grapes appearance (cystic bronchiectasis)
  - Investigation of choice: HRCT**
  - **Central Bronchiectasis is a Sign of Allergic Bronchopulmonary Aspergillosis (ABPA)****
  - **Idiopathic disease** showing tracheobronchomegaly is mounier-kuhn syndrome.

CAUSES OF CHARACTERISTIC APPEARANCES

Pulmonary lesions can be classified into:
    i. Alveolar
    ii. Interstitial.

Acinar or Alveolar Shadow

- 4-10 mm
- Coalescence
- Ill-defined
- Presence of air bronchogram (visualization of air filled bronchus due to opacification of surrounding alveoli).

Causes of Air Bronchogram** (sign given by Fleishner)

Common causes
- Pulmonary edema
- Pneumonic consolidation
- Hyaline membrane disease

Rare causes
- Contusion, hemorrhage
- Lymphoma
- Alveolar cell carcinoma
- Sarcoidosis
- ARDS
- Alveolar proteinosis.
    Note: An air bronchogram is not seen within pleural fluid and rarely within a tumour.

Collapse

Direct signs
- Displacement of fissures (MOST RELIABLE)
- Loss of aeration
- Vascular and bronchial crowding

Indirect signs: include-elevated diaphragm, mediastinal and hilar displacement and compensatory hyperinflation.

Interstitial Shadows

- Pneumoconiosis
- Sarcoidosis
- Drugs
- Collagen disorders
- Idiopathic pulmonary fibrosis.

HRCT is the Investigation of Choice**

Ground glass haze on HRCT is a sign of alveolitis signifying active and reversible stage of disease**

Important Appearances

Crazy pavement appearance characteristic of **Alveolar Proteinosis** (due to air space opacification with interlobular septal thickening)**.

Most common thoracic manifestation of rheumatoid arthritis is pleural effusion.

Egg Shell Calcification

a. Silicosis (hilar nodes)
b. Sarcoidosis
c. Treated lymphoma.

Miliary Shadowing**

Size- 2-4 mm

Causes: TB, sarcoidosis, pneumoconiosis, Histoplasmosis, chicken pox, metastasis, Alveolar microlithiasis (familial condition with multiple fine sand like calculi in alveoli), oil embolism, hemosiderosis, Histiocytosis X **.

Honey Combing

Common causes
*   Histiocytosis X.
*   Scleroderma.
*   Rheumatoid arthritis.
*   Fibrosing alveolitis.
*   Sarcoidosis.
*   Pneumoconiosis.

Rare
*   Tuberous sclerosis.
*   Gaucher's disease.
*   Lymphangiomyomatosis (seen in reproductive age group women).
*   Amyloidosis.
*   Chronic interstitial pneumonia.
*   Neurofibromatosis.

Similar appearances
- Bronchiectasis.
- Cystic fibrosis.

Caviating Lesins on CXR D/D

How to Remember
"If you see **HOLES** on chest X-ray, they are **WEIRD**":
Wegener's syndrome
Embolic (pulmonary, septic)
Infection (anaerobes, pneumocystis, TB)
Rheumatoid (necrobiotic nodules)
Developmental cysts (sequestration)
Histiocytosis
Oncological
Lymphangioleiomyomatosis
Environmental, occupational
Sarcoid.

Upper Lobe Shadowing

Breast
Beryllium
Radiation
Extrinsic allergic alveolitis
Ankylosing spondylitis
Sarcoidosis
TB
Silicosis.

HEMITHORACIC ABNORMALITY

UNILATERAL HYPERTRANSLUCENT HEMITHORAX
- Rotation—most common.
- Scoliosis.
- Poliomyelitis.
- Mastectomy.
- Polands syndrome—congenital absence pectoralis muscle.
- Pneumothorax.
- Emphysema.
- Pulmonary embolism.
- Mcleod syndrome (Swyer James syndrome).

SECTION TWO

OPAQUE HEMITHORAX
- Large pleural effusion
- Collapse, consolidation, fibrosis
- Pulmonary agenesis
- Pneumonectomy
- Thickening, mesothelioma

PULMONARY EDEMA

CLASSICALLY-"Bat wing" appearance on CXR **

Can be Cardiogenic or Non-cardiogenic due to Volume overload (renal failure) or increased capillary premeability (ARDS).

Stages of Pulmonary Edema

1. Upper lobar diversion of blood (12-19 mm Hg).
2. Interstitial edema (seen as Kerley lines) 20 mm Hg, pleural effusion.
3. Alveolar edema or the bat wing appearance seen at 25 mm Hg PCWP (Perihilar fluffy opacities).

Normal lung lymphatics are not seen but thickening of lymphatics or connective tissue produces Kerley lines.

> **Kerley A lines**-non branching lines radiating from hilum, 2-6 cm long. Thickened deep interlobular septa.
> **Kerley B lines**-transverse thin, non branching lines, 1-3 cms long ;<1mm thick at base of lung; perpendicular to pleura. They represent thick interlobular septa.
> **Kerley C lines**- spider web appearance.

Causes of Kerley Lines

- Left ventricular failure.
- Mitral stenosis.
- Pneumoconiosis.
- Lymphangitis carcinomatosis.
- Other causes include: interstitial fibrosis, sarcoidosis, alveolar cell carcinoma, lymphoma, lymphatic obstruction, lymphangiectasia, idiopathic, lymphangiomyomaosis.

Causes of ARDS

Major trauma, septicemia, shock, fat embolism, near drowning, burns, pancreatitis, Mendelson's syndrome, oxygen toxicity.

PULMONARY EMBOLISM

CXR may be normal in 30% of the patients**
Plain X-Ray signs of pulmonary embolism
- Westermark sign (area of peripheral oligaemia).
- Knuckle sign, an enlarged right descending pulmonary artery (Palla's sign).
- Hamptons hump (peripheral wedge shaped opacity with convexity towards hilum).
- Melting sign (infarct shows rapid clearing in contrast to pneumonic consolidation i.e. it melts like snow).
- Fleishner's sign, elevated hemidiaphragm.

Screening Investigation of Choice are Ventilation Perfusion Scanning and CECT

Nowadays CT is the preferred method.
V/Q Scanning**
Ventilation agents
- Xe-133
- Kr 81
- Technegas

Perfusion agents
- Tc 99 MAA (macro aggregates of albumin)
- Ventilation/perfusion mismatch is a sign of pulmonary infarct**

NORMAL VENTILATION WITH A DEFECT IN PERFUSION

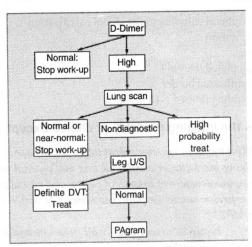

PROTOCOL FOR EVALUATION

SECTION TWO

GOLD STANDARD-PULMONARY ANGIOGRAPHY**
Latest Protocol for Evaluation of Pulmonary Embolism

If CXR is normal next investigation is V/Q scanning however is CXR is abnormal (has COPD, old lesions, etc.) where interpretation of V/Q scanning is difficult spiral CT is the next investigation recommended.

PULMONARY MALIGNANCY

Bronchogenic Carcinoma

Golden S Sign—described by Golden, Central broncho-genic carcinoma with right upper lobe collapse.**

Types (WHO Classification)

1. Squamous cell ca
2. Adeno carcinoma
3. Small cell ca
4. Large cell ca
   - *Can be divided into central & peripheral tumours*
   - *Squamous cell ca and small cell ca form central tumours while adeno carcinoma usually is a peripheral tumour***
   - *Bulky mediastanial lymphadenopathy and fastest rate of growth is characteristic of small cell ca*
   - *Squamous cell ca more likely to cavitate.*

Signs of a Malignant Solitary Pulmonary Nodule**

- Peripheral calcification or absent calcification
- Cavitation
- Size
- Spiculated margin
- Umbilicated border
- Doubling time of 1-18 months.

CT is the imaging modality of choice Except

- *MRI is useful in superior sulcus tumor and as a problem solving modality in chest wall and mediastinal invasion, involvement of branchial plexus and vasculature in superior sulcus or pancoast tumour is better seen on MRI. ***
- *MRI is better to assess chest wall invasion and hilar lymphadenopathy.*

Lung Metastasis**

Usual appearance is Cannon ball appearance they are multiple, bilateral with lower lobe predominance

Cavitating 2°—Carcinoma cervix, Squamous cell carcinoma of head and neck and Osteosarcoma

Calcifying 2°—osteosarcoma, chondrosarcoma etc mucinous carcinoma of GIT

Pneumothorax is commonly associated with metastasis from osteosarcoma**

Solitary metastasis common with colon, kidney, breast, testicular tumours, bone sarcomas and malignant melanoma.

Lymphangitis Carcinomatosa

Due to metastasis invading and occluding lymphatics
Due to:
- Lung, breast, stomach, pancreas, cervix and prostate. CXR will show reticulonodular shadowing with pleural effusions and hilar lymphadenopathy

MISCELLANEOUS

Pulmonary Hamartoma

a. POPCORN calcification**
b. Presence of fat is diagnostic of hamartoma

Radiation Injury to Chest

Earliest feature is alveolar and bronchiolar desquamation and accumulation of exudates in alveoli, followed by organization and fibrosis. Changes are remarkably geometric (corresponding to shape of the portal).

Bronchial Atresia
- More common left upper lobe.

Sequestration

A segment of lung not communicating with broncho-pulmonary tree; may communicate with foregut.

Types

1. **Intralobar** more common sequestrated segment within the same pleura.

2. **Extralobar** more involved with congenital anomalies
   Diagnostic investigation—aortography **.
   Because it has a systemic vascular supply.
   MC site is posterobasal segment of left lower lobe
   Presentation with recurrent chest infection.

CARDIOVASCULAR SYSTEM

Normal Heart

Cardiac Borders on CXR-PA View are formed by ***

   Right border—from above downwards by—Superior vena Cava, Right atrium, Inferior vena cava.

   Left border—from above downwards by—Subclavian artery, Aortic knuckle, Pulmonary artery segment, left Atrial appendage, Left ventricle.

Size

Cardiomegaly when cardiac shadow is >50% in adults and >60% in infants. **

Heart Size and Silhouette

A. **Cardiothoracic ratio**
   1. Ratio obtained by relating the largest transverse diameter of the heart to the widest internal
   2. How to measure CT ratio (see diagram)
   3. Calculation of CT ratio = (A + B) / C.

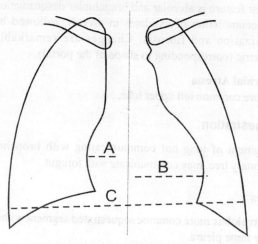

B. **Cardiac chambers diagram showing normal silhouette**

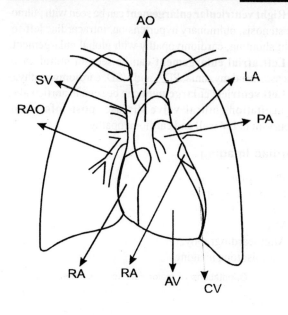

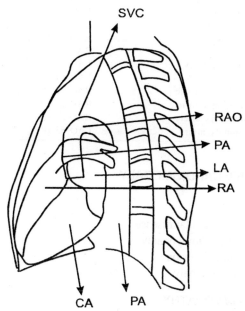

CARDIAC CHAMBER ENLARGEMENT

Right atrial enlargement can be seen with tricuspid stenosis or congenital malformation, ASD, cardiomyopathy with global enlargement.

Right ventricular enlargement can be seen with pulmonic stenosis, pulmonary hypertension, intracardiac left-to-right shunting, cardiomyopathy with global enlargement.

Left atrial enlargement can be seen in mitral valve disease, atrial myxoma, PDA and VSD, cardiomyopathy.

Left ventricle enlargement can be seen in aortic valve regurgitation, mitral valve disease, post infarction, aneurysm in LV wall and cardiomyopathy.

Cardiac Imaging

➢ Plain X-ray
➢ Echocardiography
➢ Cardiac CT
➢ MRI
➢ Angiocardiography.
➢ Radioisotope imaging.

Orientations of major cardiac structures

	Optimum projection°
Aortic arch	LAO 62 (P)
Interventricular septum	LAO 56 (E)
Interatrial septum	LAO 61 (E)
Mitral valve ring	RAO 38 (E)
Tricuspid valve ring	RAO 43 (E)
Origin right coronary	LAO 73 (P)
Origin left coronary	LAO 14 (P)
Long axis left ventricle	RAO 42 (P)
Long axis right ventricle	RAO 25 (P)
Right pulmonary artery	RAO 26 (P)
Left pulmonary artery	LAO 53 (P)

MASSIVE CARDIOMEGALY

Causes

• Multiple valvular disease
• Dilated cardiomyopathy
• Pericardial effusion
• Ebsteins anomaly

CARDIOMYOPATHY

Dilated cardiomyopathy:
➢ Cardiac enlargement (purely left ventricular or globular because of all chambers).

Hypertrophic cardiomyopathy on echocardiography.

➤ Asymmetric septal hypertrophy.
➤ Banana like left ventricular cavity.
➤ Abnormal Systolic Anterior Motion (SAM) of mitral valve.

PERICARDIUM

Congenital defect of pericardium rare; usually left sided. Causes a bulge on the left cardiac border.

Pericardial Effusion

• **Cardiomegaly with no particular chamber enlargement** **
• **Money bag or Leather bottle or flask shaped heart** with relatively clear lung fields **
• Most sensitive investigation—**echocardiography** 15 ml can be detected.

Constrictive pericarditis—MRI is the investigation done to detect thickness of pericardium; >5 mm is considered abnormal **

Restrictive cardiomyopathy is a diagnosis of exclusion *finding a normal pericardium excludes a diagnosis of constrictive pericarditis however finding of thickened pericardium doesn't necessarily imply presence of constriction.*

VALVULAR HEART DISEASE

Plain X-Ray findings of Mitral Stenosis**.
➤ Elevated left main bronchus.
➤ Carinal widening normal carinal angle is 60-75 degree.
➤ Double atrial shadow or density.
➤ Upper lobar venous diversion with prominent upper lobe veins—**stag antlers sign.**
➤ Prominent left atrial appendage (pathognomic of rheumatic heart disease) resulting in straightening of the left heart border.
➤ Barium swallow—impression on oesophagus*.
➤ **Lutembacher Syndrome**—ASD (congenital) with (acquired) MS.
➤ Long standing pulmonary venous hypertension may lead to **hemosiderosis** and ossific nodules.

MEDIASTINUM

Anterior Mediastinal Tumours (9Ts)

1. Thyroid
2. Teratoma and associated germinal cell tumors
3. Thymic tumor (thymoma associated with myasthenia gravis, pure red cell aplasia, hypogammaglobinemia)
4. Thoracic aorta and innominate artery aneurysm or tortousity.
5. Tissue tumor—bronchogenic cyst
   enteric cyst
   fibroma
   hemangioma
   lipoma or lipomatosis
   lymphadenopathy or lymphoma
   neurogenic
   pericardial lesion (pericardial cyst or spring water cyst)
6. T cell lymphoma
7. Parathyroid tumor
8. Metastasis
9. Transdiaphragmatic lesions.

Middle Mediastinal Tumours (ABCDE)

- Aneurysm of the aorta.
- Bronchogenic cyst.
- Carcinoma of the bronchus.
- Distant metastasis or lymph nodes.
- Enteric cyst.

Posterior Mediastinal Tumours

➢ Neurogenic tumor.
➢ Paravertebral abscess.
➢ Paravertebral extramedullary haemopoiesis.
➢ Paravertebral lymphoma.
➢ Paravertebral myeloma.
➢ Paravertebral metastasis.
➢ Anterior thoracic meningocele.
➢ Dilated esophagus—achalasia.
➢ Aortic aneurysm.
➢ Enteric or neuroenteric cyst.
➢ Hiatus hernia.
➢ Bochdalek hernia.

Note

Neuroenteric cyst

Developmental anomalies produced by partial or complete persistence of neuroenteric canal or its incomplete resorption. Radiological appearance—soft tissue mass in posterior mediastinum, air fluid level and vertebral anomaly as hemivertebra, butterfly vertebra or block vertebra.

CONGENITAL HEART DISEASE

The Pulmonary Vasculature

Increased pulmonary perfusion is called pulmonary plethora and is recognized by enlarged central and peripheral pulmonary arteries (Right Descending Pulmonary artery>16 mm) and veins in all zones. The pulmonary vessels in the outer third and upper zones of the lung fields are barely seen in the erect healthy patient but when there is greatly increased pulmonary perfusion, many more capillaries in these zones are recruited into the active pulmonary circulation

Decreased Pulmonary Perfusion (Oligaemia)

Pulmonary venous congestion and oedema: The diagnostic radiological features of pulmonary venous congestion and oedema in congenital heart disease are essentially the same as in acquired heart disease with both alveolar and interstitial oedema. The pattern of visible oedematous interlobular septal lines, however, tends to be different in the infant and small child; the central A lines predominate, producing a criss-cross reticular linear pattern rather than the regular costophrenic parallel horizontal Kerley B lines more frequently seen in pulmonary oedema in the adult.

Severe obstructive pulmonary arterial hypertension in congenital heart disease is due to an increased peripheral pulmonary arteriolar resistance—the Eisenmenger reaction. The central pulmonary arteries enlarge and the peripheral pulmonary arteries become smaller than normal (Peripheral Pruning).

SECTION TWO

Flow diagram of acyanotic congenital heart defects: AR, aortic regurgitation; AS, aortic stenosis; ASD, atrial septal defect; COA, coarctation of the aorta; CVH, combined ventricular hypertrophy; ECD, endocardial cushion defect; EFE, endocardial fibroelastosis; L-R, left-to-right; LVH, left ventricular hypertrophy; MR, mitral regurgitation; MS, mitral stenosis; PAPVR, partial anomalous pulmonary venous return; PBF, pulmonary blood flow; PDA, patent ductus arteriosus; PS, pulmonary stenosis; PVOD, pulmonary vascular obstructive disease (or Eisenmenger's syndrome); RBBB, right bundle branch block; RVH, right ventricular hypertrophy; VSD, ventricular septal defect.

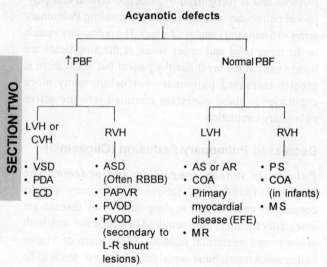

SECTION TWO

Acyanotic defects

↑ PBF

LVH or CVH
- VSD
- PDA
- ECD

RVH
- ASD (Often RBBB)
- PAPVR
- PVOD
- PVOD (secondary to L-R shunt lesions)

Normal PBF

LVH
- AS or AR
- COA
- Primary myocardial disease (EFE)
- MR

RVH
- PS
- COA (in infants)
- MS

Coarctation of Aorta

- Rib notching (inferior) involving 3-9 ribs caused by prominent intercostals collaterals, rib notching is rare before 5 years age. **
- Figure of '3' appearance of the aortic knuckle.
- Most common location is just beyond the origin of left subclavian artery.

*Flow diagram of cyanotic congenital heart defects.
CVH, combined ventricular hypertrophy; HLHS,
hypoplastic left heart syndrome; L-R, left-to-right; LVH,
left ventricular hypertrophy; PA, pulmonary artery; PBF,
pulmonary blood flow; PS, pulmonary stenosis; PVOD,
pulmonary vascular obstructive disease (or Eisenmenger's syndrome); RBBB, right bundle branch block; RV,
right ventricle; RVH, right ventricular hypertrophy;
TAPVR, total anomalous pulmonary venous return; TGA,
transposition of the great arteries; TOF, tetralogy of
fallot; VSD, ventricular septal defect.*

Cyanotic defects

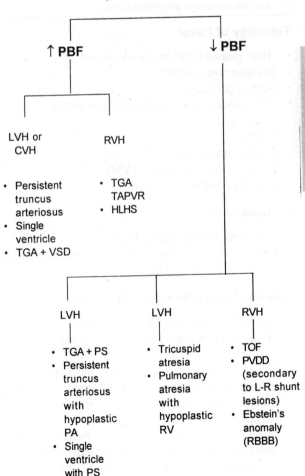

SECTION TWO

Causes of Rib Notching

RIB Notching
Inferior surface of ribs

Bilateral
- Coarctation, aortic thrombosis, subclavian obstruction
- SVC/IVC obstruction (Rare)
- Pulmonary AV malformation, intercostals pulmonary fistula
- Neurogenic, hyperparathyroidism

Unilateral
- Balock-taussing operation
- Subclavian artery occlusion

Superior rib notching
- Connective tissue disorders—RA, SLE, scleroderma, etc.
- Hyperparathyroidism
- Marfans syndrome, poliomyelitis etc.

Tetralogy of Fallot

- 'Boot shaped heart' or cor-en sabot**
- Pulmonary oligaemia *
- Normal size heart.
- 25% association with right sided aortic arch
  Components of tetralogy are:
  1. VSD
  2. Infundibular stenosis
  3. Aortic root over rides the VSD
  4. Right ventricular hypertrophy.

Ebsteins Anomaly

- Atrialization of the right ventricle
- CXR massive globular cardiomegaly with pulmonary oligaemia. Box shaped heart.

Cyanotic Heart Diseases with Plethora

TGA (most common), TAPVC, truncus arteriosus.
Total Anomalous Pulmonary Venous Drainage (TAPVC)
**

- Three types supracardiac, cardiac or infracardiac
- Snowman appearance or Figure of 8 appearance—seen in supracardiac type of TAPVC (because of large ascending vein on the left side)
- Remember—in obstructive TAPVC, there is a normal sized heart with severe pulmonary venous hypertension resulting in "ground glass" appearance of the lungs.

- Scimitar Syndrome: Partial anomalous pulmonary venous connection with right lower lobe vein draining below diaphragm into systemic circulation and hypoplasia of right lower lobe and dextroposition of heart**.

Transposition of Great Arteries (TGA)

D-TGA or uncorrected TGA
- Egg on side appearance **
- Enlarged, rounded heart with pulmonary plethora and a narrow pedicle

Corrected TGA or L-TGA
- Long smooth curve to the left heart border, water fall appearance.

L-R Shunt (VSD, PDA)

- Most common type of VSD is perimembranous
- Pulmonary plethora
- Only diagnosed on X-Ray as cardiomegaly or plethora if shunt is >2:1 (ratio of pulmonary to systemic flow)

ASD

- Types ostium primum defects and ostium secundum defects Ostium secundum is more common.
- Hilar dance on fluoroscopy **
- Primum defect is seen in Downs syndrome.

Patent Ductus Arteriosus

- Best echocardiographic view to demonstrate PDA is parasternal short axis view
- On X-ray may show calcification of ductus or bump in the aortic contour

Pulmonary Arterial Hypertension

Characteristic appearance is that of a large main and large central pulmonary arteries which taper down rapidly to very small vessels over a few order of branches, giving a '**pruned tree** appearance'. Calcification may be seen in long standing pulmonary hypertension.

Eisenmenger syndrome: Development of irreversible pulmonary damage leads to reversal of shunt, which may "paradoxically show apparent improvement" of the CXR appearance.

SECTION TWO

Pulmonary Arteriovenous Malformations

➢ Usually associated with **osler-weber-rendu syndrome**
➢ Act as a right to left shunt

Klippel Trenaunay Syndrome

• Nevus with hypertrophy of soft tissue and bones of the affected limb. There is venous dysplasia with persistence of primitive venous system.

RADIOISOTOPES IN CARDIAC IMAGING

Ischaemic Heart Disease

Thallium 201-**infarct–Cold spot on thallium perfusion scanning****

Reversible ischaemia will be cold on exercise and normal on rest while irreversible infarct will be cold on both. So thallium determines the reversibility of a lesion. **

Tc^{99} **pyrophosphate**—infarct binding agent (infarct scintigraphy)–hot spot on scanning***.

Functional Isotope Imaging in Heart

To evaluate ventricular function can be done by two methods first pass method and gated equilibrium studies, gated studies are also known as multiple gated acquisition (MUGA).

AORTA

• Investigation of choice for aortic dissection is MRI ***
• Aorto-arteritis most commonly involves the subclavian vessels and next most commonly the renal vessels.**
• Most common site for aortic injury is aortic isthmus just distal to left subclavian artery.**
• Most common variant of aortic arch anatomy is common origin of innonimate and left common carotid.
• Sinus of valsalva aneurysm rupture into right sided cardiac chambers creating a left to right shunt.

CARDIAC TUMOURS

• Most common is secondary involvement from breast or bronchus tumours.
• Most common primary tumour heart is **myxoma**.

SKELETAL SYSTEM
Congenital Disorders/Syndromes

Associations of Absent Radius

- Ectodermal dysplasia
- Holt-Oram syndrome
- Fanconi anaemia
- Thrombocytopenia—absent radius (TAR) syndrome
- Trisomy 18
- Thalidomide embryopathy
- Renal, ear and esophageal anomalies.

   How to remember—THEFT,

T-TAR syndrome,
H-holt-oram,
E-ectodermal dysplasia,
F-Fanconi anemia,
T-trisomy/thalidomide.

Achondroplasia

- Autosomal dominant with rhizomelic dwarfism (short-ening of the proximal bones like femur and humerus)
- Narrow sacrosciatic notch leading to **champagne glass** pelvic inlet**
- **Trident hand** with short stubby fingers—fingers diverge from each other in two pairs plus thumb
- *Chevron sign* or ball and socket epiphysometaphyseal junction**
- Lumbar canal stenosis
- Bullet nose vertebrae
- *Posterior scalloping of vertebra* (also in Neuro-fibromatosis, spinal tumours, Acromegaly)**
- Most common cause of *disproportionate dwarfism*
- *Tombstone* stone *iliac blades* with posteriorly set acetabulum
- Small sella.

Mucopolysaccharidosis

- Type 1 hurlers, Type IV morquios.
- Oar shaped ribs.
- Anterior beaking of vertebrae central in morquios and anteroinferior in hurlers**.

SECTION TWO

- J- Shaped sella (due to prominent sulcus chiasmaticus also seen in 5% normal population, optic chiasm Glioma) **
- Proximal tapering of metacarpals
- Platyspondyly
- Simian pelvis.

Cleidocranial Dysplasia

Benign hereditary condition which shows:
- Partial or complete absence of clavicles, narrow thorax, wormian bones and defective ossification of pubis.

Pyknodysostosis

Characteristic features are:
- Increased bone density
- Spool shaped vertebrae
- Obtuse angle mandible.

Osteogenesis Imperfecta

- Characterized by increased bone fragility, osteoporosis and dental abnormality.
- Abnormality of type I collagen.
- **Sillence classification** four types out of which type II is lethal *in utero.*
- **Differentiated from Battered baby syndrome** in battered baby fractures are Metaphyseal while in osteogenesis imperfecta they are diaphyseal.

Osteopetrosis

- Generalized increase in bone density
- Bone within bone appearance
- Erlenmeyer flask deformity femur
- **'Rugger jersey' spine, spondylolisthesis**

Meloreosteosis (leri's disease)

- Molten candle wax appearance.**

Nail Patella Syndrome

- Iliac horns
- Hypoplastic patella/dislocation patella
- Capitulum abnormalities.

Thanatophoric Dwarfism**

- Most common fatal neonatal dysplasia
- H-shaped vertebrae
- **Telephone handle long bones**
- Clover leaf skull.

CHROMOSOMAL DISORDERS

Downs Syndrome

- Brachycephaly
- Hypoplasia of nasal, maxilla and sphenoids
- Clinodactyly
- Absent frontal sinus
- Atlantoaxial instability
- Iliac index<60
- 11 pair ribs
- Duodenal atresia, Hirschsprung disease
- Endocardial cushion defect in heart
- Aberrant right subclavian artery
- Double manubrium centers
- Hypoteleorism
- Lumbar vertebrae greater in height than width
- Increase nuchal fold thickness in first trimester >3 mm abnormal
- Short femur and short humerus
- Hydronephrosis
- Single umbilical artery
- Choroids plexus cysts
- Cerebral ventriculomegaly
- Non immune hydrops
- Cholecystomegaly
- Microcolon, echogenic small bowel
- Transient myeloproliferative disorder of infancy.

Ultrasound markers of Down's Syndrome/Trisomy 21
1. As many as 80% of infants with Down's syndrome have redundant skin in the posterior part of neck (NUCHAL TRANSLUCENCY).
   - Typically measured in 10-14 weeks
   - A measurement of 3 mm or more is taken as abnormal
2. Echogenic cardiac foci or echogenic chordae tendinae seen in 39% of trisomy 13 and 18% of fetuses with trisomy 21.

3. Echogenic bowel is seen in 10% of fetuses with trisomy 21.
4. Choroid plexus cysts are seen in 50% of fetuses with trisomy 18.

Association of Cystic Hygroma

- Turner syndrome.
- Noonan syndrome.
- Fetal alcohol syndrome.
- Nuchal bleb syndrome.

Trisomy 13 (Patau Syndrome)

- Holoprosencephaly.
- Anophthalmia .
- Congenital heart defect, e.g. VSD, ASD, PDA, dextrocardia.
- Ventral wall defect.
- Cystic kidneys.
- Polydactyly.
- Mid line facial anomalies.
- Cutis aplasia in parieto-occipital area.

Trisomy 18 (Edward Syndrome)

- IUGR and polyhydramnios.
- Clenched hand with overlapping index finger.
- Rockerbottom /club feet.
- Forearm anomalies—radial ray defects.
- Omphalocele.
- Diaphragmatic hernias.
- Horseshoe kidney.
- Congenital heart disease.
- Colonic mal rotation.
- Myelomeningocele.
- Brain and vertebral anomalies.
- Hypospadias .
- Cryptorchidism.

ENDOCRINE DISORDERS

Cretinism

- Delayed skeletal and dental maturity**
- Stippled epiphysis or epiphyseal dysgenesis **
- Cherry or bowl shaped sella.

Acromegaly

- Prognathism**
- Increased heel pad thickness (normal 21mm in females and 23 mm in males)
- Hyper pneumatization of sinuses**
- Ballooned sella
- Prominent muscular markings
- Widened joint spaces and premature osteoarthritis
- Tufted distal phalanges.

CHARACTERISTIC RADIOLOGICAL APPEARANCES

Anterior Scalloping of Vertebrae

- Aortic aneurysm.
- Lymphadenopathy.
- Subperiosteal TB.
- Down's syndrome.

Posterior Scalloping

- Achondroplasia.
- Neurofibromatosis.
- Spinal cord tumour.
- Dural ectasia.
- Acromegaly.

Wormian Bones

- Osteogenesis imperfecta.
- Down's syndrome.
- Cretinism.
- Cleidocranial dysplasia.

Causes of Generalized Increased Bone Density**

- Renal osteodystrophy.
- Flourosis.
- Mastocytosis.
- Sclerotic metastasis.
- Osteopetrosis (Marble bone disease).
- Myeloid metaplasia.

Resorption of Lateral End of Clavicles

- Rheumatoid arthritis.
- Hyperparathyroidism.
- Multiple myeloma.
- Cleidocranial dysplasia.
- Pyknodysostosis.

Ivory Vertebra**

- Lymphoma.
- Infection.
- Metastasis.
- Pagets disease.

Madelung's Deformity

- Common in girls, usually bilateral.
- Defective development of the inner third of the epiphysis of the lower end radius resulting in bayonet like deformity on lateral view.
- Associated with Leri-Weil syndrome, Turner's syndrome, trauma, infection.

Congenital Dislocation Hip

Ultrasound should be used as initial imaging as it can visualize the cartilaginous femoral head.

Pseudoarthosis of Tibia and Fibula

Causes:
- Neurofibromatosis.
- Fibrous dysplasia.
- Idiopathic juvenile osteoporosis.

Vertebrae Plana

- Metastasis/Melanoma.
- Eosinophilic granuloma.
- Lymphoma.
- Trauma/Tuberculosis.

(How to Remember-Melt)

Normal Metacarpal Index

- 5.4-7.9.
- 8.4-10 = ARACHNODACTYLY.
- Seen in Marfan's syndrome, Homocystinuria.

Widened Intercondylar Notch Knee

- **Classically seen in Hemophilic arthopathy****
- Also in TB, JRA.
- Most common joint involved in hemophilia is knee involvement is frequently bilateral, wide and deep intercondylar notch. Patella has rectangular shape.

I/V Disc Calcification

- Idiopathic.
- Posttraumatic.
- Ochronosis.
- Ankylosing spondylitis.

Bare Orbit Sign**

- Neurofibromatosis**
- Metastasis
- Meningioma.

Short Fourth Metacarpal (Metacarpal sign)

- Turner's syndrome.
- Pseudohypoparathyroidism.

METABOLIC AND HEMATOLOGICAL DISORDERS

Hyperparathyroidism

Subperiosteal resorption is the hallmark**
Subperiosteal resorption is best seen on radial aspect of middle phalanx of 2nd and 3rd fingers**

Loss of lamina dura of teeth**.

Intracortical bone resorption—Pepper-pot skull or salt and pepper skull. Also basket work appearance of cortex

Brown tumors locally destructive areas of intense osteoclastic activity-commonly affects mandible**

Commonly due to **parathyroid adenoma.** Localized by **thallium Tc subtraction scanning or by using sestamibi scanning****

Soft tissue and vascular calcification is the hallmark of secondary hyperparathyroidism; while chondrocalcinosis is seen in primary form**

Rickets**

- Earliest—Loss of provisional zone of calcification.
- Cupping, fraying and splaying.
- Widening of growth plate.
- Healing shown by appearance of **white line of healing**
- Differential diagnosis—Metaphyseal dysplasia.

Osteomalacia

- Hallmark is presence of Looser's zones or pseudo-fractures**.

Sites:
- Pubic ramii, neck of femur, ribs, lateral border scapula Biconcave vertebrae.
- Triradiate pelvis.
- Biconcave vertebral bodies (cod fish vertebrae).

Scurvy**

Rare before 6 months of age since the storage of vitamin C in neonate is generally adequate.
- **Wimberger sign:** presence of a sclerotic rim around epiphysis.
- **White line of frankel:** dense zone of provisional calcification at the growing metaphysis.
- **Trumerfeld zone:** a lucent zone below white line due to lack of mineralisation.
- **Pelkan spur:** as the area is prone to fractures manifesting at cortical margin.
- Osteoporosis.
- Subperiosteal haemorrhage.

Renal Osteodystrophy **

- A combination of osteosclerosis, osteomalacia and secondary hyperparathyroidism.
- Rugger jersey spine due to sclerosis at the vertebral endplates.
- Rotting fence post appearance at the femoral neck.
- Increase bone density.

Osteoporosis Measurement of Bone Mass

Several noninvasive techniques are now available for estimating skeletal mass or density. These include dual-energy X-ray absorptiometry (DXA), single-energy X-ray absorptiometry (SXA), quantitative computed tomography (CT), and ultrasound.

DEXA is a highly accurate X-ray technique that has become the standard for measuring bone density in most centers. Though it can be used for measurements of any skeletal site, clinical determinations are usually made of the lumbar spine and hip. Portable DXA machines have been developed that measure the heel (calcaneus), forearm (radius and ulna), or finger (phalanges), and DXA can also be used to measure body composition. In the DXA technique, two X-ray energies are used to estimate the area of mineralized tissue, and the mineral content is divided by the area, which partially corrects for body size.

CT is used primarily to measure the spine, and peripheral CT is used to measure bone in the forearm or tibia. Research into the use of CT for measurement of the hip is ongoing. The results obtained from CT are different from all others currently available since this technique specifically analyzes trabecular bone and can provide a true density (mass of bone per unit volume) measurement. However, CT remains expensive, involves greater radiation exposure, and is less reproducible.

SECTION TWO

Hemolytic Anemia

Thalassemia

- Diploic widening (sparing the occipit) with **Hair on end or crew cut or hair-brush** appearance.
- Widening of short bones of hands **(earliest change)****
- **Flask shaped femora.**
- **Rodent facies** due to obliteration of paranasal air sinuses because of marrow hyperplasia.

Sickle Cell Anemia**

- Medullary infarcts**
- H-shaped vertebrae due to vertebral body infarcts
- Bone within bone appearance** (also in osteopetrosis)
- Salmonella osteomyelitis**
- Autosplenectomy.**

Leukemia

• Most characteristic sign is presence of Metaphyseal translucencies (occurring in 90% of cases).

Pagets Disease**

• Picture frame vertebrae.
• Cotton wool skull.
• Osteoporosis circumscripta (seen in early stage).

Rugger Jersey Spine**

• Osteopetrosis.
• Renal osteodystrophy.

Erlenmeyer Flask Deformity

• Metaphyseal dysplasia (Pyles disease).
• Thalassemia.
• Osteopetrosis.
• Gaucher's disease etc.

Gout

Features:
• Erosions usually involve cortex than articular surface due to deposition of sodium biurate.
• Tophi or eccentric soft tissue swelling.

OSTEOCHONDRITIS

AVASCULAR NECROSIS: MR scanning is the most sensitive and specific means of detecting changes in avascular necrosis, sensitivity and specificity around 100%.

PERTHES DISEASE

• Flattened and dense femoral capital epiphysis**.
• Waldenstrom sign-lateral displacement of the femoral head.
• Subcortical fissures.
• Classification on the basis of presence of sequestrum, Metaphyseal reaction and subchondral fractures known as CATTERALL CLASSIFICATION.

Infarction

- Proximal femoral epiphysis—Perthe's.
- Distal epiphysis of 2nd metatarsal—Freiberg's.
- Navicular—Kohler's.
- Lunate—Kienbock's.

Traction Injury

- Tibial tubercle: Osgood Schlatter's.
- Distal pole of patella—Sinding Larsen's.
- Os calcis: Sever's.
- Ring epiphysis of vertebral body- Scheurmann's.
- Capitulum: Panner's.
- Scaphoid: Preoser's.
  Transchordal fractures: Osteochondritis dissecans.

INFECTIONS

Osteomyelitis

- EARLIEST: soft tissue swelling and loss of soft tissue planes**.
- Bone Destruction—10-14 days.
- **Involucrum**—3 weeks.
- **Sequestrum**—4 weeks (Dead-dense bone).
- **Cloace.**

Using bone scanning diagnosis of osteomyelitis can be confirmed as early as 48 hours after disease onset.

MRI demonstrates OM as early as bone scan and is the investigation of choice when available.

Brodie's abscess: Well circumscribed area of destruction with surrounding sclerosis showing finger like extension into neighbouring bone called as **tunneling which is pathognomic.**

Tuberculosis of bone is characterized by osteoporosis and lack of periosteal reaction and less new bone formation.

Tuberculosis of spine is commonly Paradiscal type so is characterized by disc space narrowing, collapse of vertebrae and large paravertebral abscess.

Leprosy

- Licked candy stick appearance due to neuropathic resorption of bone.

Mycetoma (Madura foot)

Shaggy periostitis, reactive sclerosis 'melting snow appearance'.

Congenital Syphilis**

- Wimberger sign: erosion of the medial upper tibial metaphysis.
- **Periostitis**—Most common feature leads to cortical thickening known as **Saber Tibia***.
- Hot Cross Bun Skull**.
- Hutchison teeth, mulberry molar.
- Deafness.
  Syphilis of the skull vault: moth eaten appearance skull.

Congenital Rubella

- Celery stalk appearance.**

ARTHRITIS

Osteoarthritis

Signs (How to Remember).

Loss

Loss of joint space.
Osteopyhtes.
Subchondral sclerosis.
Subchondral cysts.

- Shows Bouchard (PIP) and Heberden Nodes (DIP).* (**HOW TO REMEMBER**—B comes before H alphabetically so Bouchard nodes occur in proximal joints while Heberden nodes in Distal joints).
- Bone most commonly involved in osteoarthritis is **patella.**

Rheumatoid Arthritis

- Earliest appearance is periarticular soft tissue swelling**.
- Then, juxta articular osteoporosis.
- Subchondral erosions (view to detect erosions **Ball Catcher's view**).
- Most commonly joints involved are carpals, metacarpophalangeal and proximal interphalangeal joints**

- Deformities—ulnar deviation of hand and fingers, swan neck deformity, Boutonniere deformity, hallux valgus, hammer toe.**
- **Juvenile rheumatoid arthritis** is characterized by epiphyseal enlargement, erosions, and periostitis.
- Cervical spine involvement is common in rheumatoid arthritis.

Psoriasis

- Most commonly involves **DIP (distal interphalangeal joints)**.
- **Cup-and-pencil** appearance.
- Sausage digit (periostitis with soft tissue swelling).
- Normal bone density.
- Opera glass hand.
- Paravertebral ossification.

Ankylosing Spondylitis

- Bamboo spine.
- Romanus sign.
- Squaring of vertebrae (due to anterior longitudinal ligament ossification).
- Calcification of I/V disc.
- Dagger sign.
- Enthesopathy.
- Symmetric sacroileitis initially more on the iliac side.

TUMOURS (Fig 2.4)

GENERAL PRINCIPLES OF RADIOLOGICAL DIAGNOSIS OF BONE TUMOURS

1. Is the lesion single or multiple?
2. What type of bone is involved?
3. Where is the lesion within the bone?
4. Radiographic features?
5. Margins of the lesion?

Osteosarcoma

- Codmans triangle**.
- Sunray appearance**.
- Can be seen secondary to Paget's disease, infarct, chronic OM, radiation exposure, diaphyseal aclasia etc
- Metaphyseal, around knee.

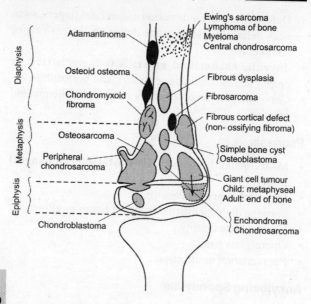

Fig. 2.4: Sites of origin of primary bone neoplasms

- *Myositis ossificans vs parosteal osteosarcoma*: Myositis differentiates from periphery while osteosarcoma from center.**
- Pulmonary metastasis have a high incidence of Pneumothorax.
- Following X-rays, prime investigation to be done is MRI.
- Parosteal osteosarcoma—occurs commonly in posterior distal femur and proximal humerus; show a radiolucent zone between tumour and underlying bone.

Osteoblastoma

Majority of the lesions occur in spine and flat bones, show an area of radiolucency around 2-10 cm.

Ewings Sarcoma

- Onion peel appearance.
- Soft tissue extension.
- Diaphyseal in location.

Chondrosarcoma

1. Primary.
2. Secondary.

Can arise from osteochondroma (1% risk) or from diaphyseal aclasia (multiple osteochondromas (10% risk). Or from chondromas.

Chondromas

- MC site is phalanges**.
- Radiological appearance—"O ring sign", may show pathognomic "pop-corn "or annular calcification.
- **Associated syndromes:**
  1. **Ollier's disease:** multiple enchondromas.
  2. **Maffuci's disease:** multiple enchondromas with haemangiomas, risk of malignant change (chondrosarcoma) is 20%.

Chondroblastoma

Usually occurs in the epiphysis or apophysis

Simple Bone Cyst (unicameral bone cyst)

- Majority in proximal humerus and femur, show an area of translucency in meta-diaphysis.
- Signs because of a pathological fracture in the lesion are:
  1. Fallen fragment sign.
  2. Trap door sign.

Giant Cell Tumour or Osteoclastoma

- Soap bubble appearance, around knee and lower end radius.
- Subarticular, eccentric lytic lesion is classical appearance.
- D/D from aneurysmal bone cyst—¾ of the aneurysmal bone cysts occur before epiphyseal closure.

Fibrous Cortical Defect

- MC site distal posteromedial femoral cortex. Seen as blister like expansion of the cortex with thin shell of overlying bone.

Adamantinoma

- Unusual tumour invariably located in tibial shaft, histologically has epithelial derivation.
- Radiologically appears as an eccentric area of destruction involving the anterior portion of tibial shaft.

Chordoma

- Usually purely lytic, with evidence of calcification, common in sacrum and /or coccyx and basi-occipit and basi-spenoid.

Fibrous Dysplasia

1. Monosteotic.
2. Polyosteotic.

Features

- Ground glass appearance on X-Ray**.
- Shepherd Crook deformity femur**.
- Leonine facies.
- **Mcalbright syndrome**—polyosteotic fibrous dysplasia with precocious puberty.
- Increased uptake on radionuclide scanning.

Haemangioma

- Common in vertebrae, particularly lumbar.
- **On plain X-Ray vertical striations or Codruy Cloth appearance**.
- On CT: **Polka dot appearance**.
- High signal on both T1 andT2 WI on MRI.

Vanishing Bone Disease

- Gorham's disease.
- Angiomatosis of the bone.**

Myeloma Vs Metastasis

- Multiple myeloma shows classical Rain Drop appearance (due to punched out lytic lesions skull).
- Metastatis characteristically involve **pedicle.**
- **Mandible** is more commonly involved in multiple myeloma.
- Alkaline phosphatase is normal in myeloma.
- For multiple myeloma skeletal survey is better than scintigraphy because it is essentially osteolytic with no bone reaction.

Sclerotic Metastasis**

- Prostate.
- Stomach.
- Carcinoid.

Lytic Expansile Metastasis**

- Renal cell ca.
- Thyroid.

Skeletal Metastases—Common Radiological Appearance

Lung.
Carcinoma-lytic.
Carcinoid-sclerotic.
Breast-lytic or mixed.
Genitourinary.
Renal cell carcinoma-lytic, expansile.
Wilms tumour-lytic.
Bladder (TCC)-lytic, occasionally sclerotic
Prostate-sclerotic.

Reproductive organs.
Cervix-lytic or mixed.
Uterus-lytic.
Ovary-lytic.
Testes-lytic; occasionally sclerotic.

Thyroid.
Lytic, expansile.

GIT.
Stomach-sclerotic or mixed.
Colon-lytic; occasionally sclerotic.
Rectum-lytic.

Adrenal
Phaechromocytoma- Lytic, expansile.
Carcinoma-lytic.
Neuroblastoma- lytic; occasionally sclerotic.

Skin
Squamous cell carcinoma-lytic.
Melanoma-lytic, expansile.

SECTION TWO

TRAUMA

Open Fracture

Radiographic signs:
- Protusion of bone fragments beyond soft tissue margins.
- Subcutaneous gas.
- Absebce of parts of bone or soft tissue disruption.
- Presence of Foreign material.

Neuropathic Joints or Charcot's Joints

Causes
- Diabetes, leprosy, syringomyelia, neurosyphilis, spina bifida etc.

X-ray appearance

5-D's

Disorganization.

Increased bone **D**ensity.

Debris within joint capsule.

Destruction.

Deformity.

Shoulder Dislocation

Most commonly **anteriorly**

Defect in posterior superior aspect of humeral HATCHET OR HILL-SACH'S DEFORMITY.

Injury to inferior portion of glenoid-bankart's lesion.

Posterior dislocation: persistent internal rotation of humerus-LIGHT BULB appearance.

Inferior dislocation or luxatio erecta—arm is locked in abduction.

Terry Thomas Sign

- Scapholunate dislocation.

Spondylolisthesis**

- **Inverted napolean hat sign** on AP view.
- Beheaded Scottish terrier sign on oblique view.
- Normal oblique view shows Scotty dog appearance.
- Scotty dog wearing a collar in spondylolysis.

GASTROINTESTINAL TRACT

SALIVARY GLANDS

- Three-fourths of the salivary gland tumours are pleomorphic adenomas. Show calcification.
- Warthin's or adenolymphoma appear hot on radio-nuclide scan.
- **Adenoid cystic tumour show perineural invasion.**

ESOPHAGUS

Dysphagia

Barium is better for evaluation of motility disorders and for cricopharyngeal dysphagia than endoscopic evaluation (if dysphagia is more to liquids than to solids).

Achalasia Cardia**

- Dilated sigmoid esophagus.
- Rat tailed or bird beak tapering**
- Precipated by methylcholine.
- Obstruction relived by amyl nitrate, hot water.
- Premalignant condition.

Corkscrew Oesophagus

- Diffuse oesophageal spasm.

Carcinoma Esophagus

Barium study will show:
- Irregular narrowing.
- Mucosal destruction.
- Shouldered margins.

   Role of CT and endoscopic USG for staging of tumour and for diagnosis use endoscopy and biopsy.

Scleroderma

Commonly affects the esophagus (lower 2/3rd) with wide open GE junction and GE reflux.

Diaphragmatic Hernia

- Most common diaphragmatic hernia is hiatus hernia; other are Bochdalek's hernia more common left side, posteriorly and due to patent pleuro-peritoneal canals

and Morgani's hernia due to defect between sternal and costal part of diaphragm, it is anterior and more common on right side.
- Bochdalek's hernia may show 13 pair of ribs (most common congenital diaphragmatic hernia)
- Post traumatic hernia on barium study will show a bowel loop hernaiting into thorax through a narrow diaphragmatic tear—**love bird sign.**

Hiatus Hernia

Diagnostic criteria on barium study:
- GE Junction is >2 cm above hiatus.
- Hiatus is >2.5 cm.
- More than 3 gastric folds extend above the Hiatus.
  GE junction is normal in Rolling or Para esophageal hernia.

STOMACH AND DUODENUM

Hypertrophic Pyloric Stenosis**
- Initial investigation is USG
- Criteria US-size of Pylorus Greater than 14C17 mm, >4 mm wall thickness
- **Barium-signs**
  1. String sign
  2. Shouldering
  3. Apple core appearance
  4. Double track sign
  5. Beak sign.

Ulcer Disease (Fig. 2.5)

Double contrast barium examination preferred to single contrast examination.

Benign vs. Malignant Ulcer

Location lesser curvature more likely benign and greater curvature likely malignant.
- Benign ulcers are most commonly seen along lesser curvature and adjacent part of posterior wall; geriatic or old age ulcers occur high in lesser curve, aspirin or drug ulcers occur in dependent part of greater curve. Benign ulcer is rare high on greater curvature, so it is a suspicious location for malignancy.

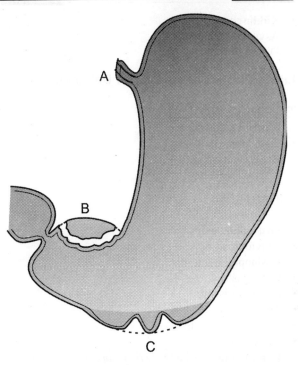

Fig. 2.5: Three characteristic types of gastric ulcer; the shading represents barium. **A.** benign, projecting, lesser curvature ulcer with collar (broken lines) **B.** Malignant, intraluminal ulcer with irregular ulcer with irregular nodular tumor rim; **C.** Non projecting benign greater curvature ulcer

Signs of Benign Ulcer

- Hamptom's line-overhanging mucosa at the margins of a benign ulcer.
- Crescent sign.
- Projecting beyond the contour of the stomach.
- Response to medical therapy.
- Folds reaching upto the edge of ulcer-spoke wheel pattern.
- Normal peristalsis.

Malignant Ulcer

- Carmanns meniscus sign-margin of the ulcerating tumour projects into the gastric lumen.

- Kirklin complex**
- Asymmetric mound
- Distorted folds.

Linitis Plastica or the Leather Bottle Stomach

THE ENTIRE STOMACH
- Gastric carcinoma
- Hodgkins lymphoma
- Breast metastasis
- Kaposis sarcoma

THE ANTRUM
- Corrosives
- Post radiotherapy
- Amyloidosis
- Eosinophilic enteritis
- CMV gastritis
- Crohn's disease
- TB
- Secondary syphilis
- Sarcoidosis.

Lymphoma *is more likely than carcinoma when there is extensive wall thickening; circumferential involvement of stomach, transpyloric spread is there, presence of lymph nodes above and below renal hilum and splenomegaly.*

Bull's Eye Lesion in Stomach

- Submucosal metastatis (most common melanoma) **
- Lymphoma
- Carcinoma breast, bronchus, pancreas
- Carcinoid
- Leiomyoma
- Pancreatic rests, neurofibroma.

Trifoliate Duodenum (on Barium meal)

- Chronic duodenal ulcer with scarring.

Constriction of Transverse Duodenum

- Superior mesenteric artery syndrome.

Double Bubble Appearance

- Duodenal atresia.
- Annular pancreas.

Duodenal Webs

Wind-sock like appearance (an intraluminal diverticulum)
Triple bubble- jejunal atresia.

SMALL AND LARGE BOWEL

Malabsorption**

Radiological Signs**
- Bowel loop dilatation.
- Intestinal hurry.
- Flocculation of contrast—snow flake like deposit on the mucosa.
- Segmentation.
- Fold thickening.
- Excessive secretion/dilution of contrast.
- Moulage sign: tube like appearance of bowel.

Intraperitoneal Fluid

Hellmer's Sign: lucent band between liver and lateral abdominal wall due to ascitis.

Ascariasis

Various signs have been described for ascariasis which include "sphagetti appearance", "bulls eye sign" and "impacted worm sign". The 'inner tube" or the "double tube" signs imply the visualisation of the hypoechoic alimentary canal seen within the round cross section of the worm. On a plain X-ray **medusa head appearance** has been described.

Ileocaecal Kochs

Named signs
- "String sign".
- Fleishner or inverted umbrella sign due to thickened and gaping ileocaecal valve with narrow terminal ileum.
- Sterlein sign.
- Gooseneck appearance-ileum hanging from fibrosed, pulled up caecum.
- Purse string appearance.

SECTION TWO

String Sign in Radiology
Seen in
- Crohn's disease
- Tuberculosis
- Hypertrophic pyloric stenosis.

Ulcerative Colitis

- *Toxic Megacolon* if transverse colon >5.5 cm
- Collar button ulcers.
- Pseudopolyps.
- Contiguous, mucosal involvement.
- Reflux ileitis.
- Pipe sem colon (ahaustral).
- Increased presacral space normally its <1 cm.
- Risk of malignant change higher than Crohn's.
- Blurring of mucosal stripe and granular appearance is the earliest sign.*
- If suspecting active disease an instant barium enema can be done which is done without preparation as actively inflamed colon is almost always free of fecal matter.

Crohn's Disease

- Skip lesions.
- Transmural involvement.
- HALO SIGN on CT.
- String sign of kantor.
- Cobble stone appearance.
- Raspberry/rose thorn appearance.
- Strictures and fistulae more common.
- Pseudosacculations.
- Earliest change is–apthoid ulceration. *

Stacked Coin Appearance

- Due to Submucosal hemorrhages like seen in Henoch-scolein purpura.

Scalloped Edges of Sigmoid Colon

- Pneumatosis intestinalis (submucosal air cysts).

Saw Tooth Appearance

- Diverticulosis.
- MC site sigmoid colon.
- Concertina-like or serrated appearance

Congenital Abdominal Wall Defects

Omphalocele

- Umbilical cord is normal in position.
- Liver is a common component.
- Bound by a membrane.
- Associated chromosomal anomalies common.

Gastroshchisis

- Bowel loops are seen free floating in the amniotic cavity.
- Defect is located in right paraumbilical region.
- Bowel complications common.

Hirschsprung Disease

- Barium is diluted in saline not water to prevent water intoxication from absorption in megacolon.
- **Most important sign on barium enema is sudden change of caliber from narrow aganglionic segment and dilated proximal bowel.**

ACUTE ABDOMEN

Perforation

- Best projection to demonstrate pnemoperitoneum—**CXR****.
- If the patient cannot get into an erect position then Left Lateral Decubitus Projection is required**.
- Patient should be in that position for **10 min** at least for air to rise up.
- By careful technique even 1 ml of free air can be detected.

Supine Film Signs of Pneumoperitoneum **

- **Football sign**—collection of air in the center of the abdomen over a fluid collection.
- Riglers sign (visualization of both aspects of bowel wall being outlined by air on either side).
- **Cupola sign**—large amount of gas under the diaphragm
- Falciform ligament, inverted V sign.
- **Triangle sign**—Air between bowel loop.
  Chilladiti syndrome or interposition of colon between liver and diaphragm can mimic pneumoperitoneum.**

Other Causes of Pseudopneumoperitoneum

- Subdiaphragmatic fat.
- Pulmonary collapse.
- Omental fat.
- Subphrenic abscess etc.
- Uneven diaphragm.
- Subpulmonary pneumothorax etc.

Intestinal Obstruction

Small Bowel Obstruction

- Multiple centrally placed loops with valvulae connvinates in jejunum and diameter 3-5 cm.
- May show **String of beads** appearance due to air trapped within valvulae and rest of loop being fluid filled.

Large Bowel Obstruction

- Few peripherally placed loops with haustrae and diameter 5 cm + and showing fecal matter within dilated loop.
- A caecal diameter of >9 cm implies impending perforation. **
- Demonstration of the air in rectum implies a paralytic ileus rather than mechanical obstruction.**

> String of beads in radiology
> —Fibromuscular dysplasia
> —Chr. Pancreatitis (chain of lakes)
> —Small bowel obstruction.

Intususception**

Radiological Signs
- Coiled spring appearance.
- Claw sign.
- Empty right iliac fossa.
- Barium enema can be both diagnostic and therapeuptic
- Can use pneumatic reduction.
- "Double target appearance" on X-ray and USG.

Coffee Bean Sign

- Strangulation of incompletely obstructed loop of small intestine.

Sigmoid Volvulus**

Signs
- Liver overlap sign.
- Left flank overlap sign.
- Apex below left hemi diaphragm.
- Inferior convergence on the left.
- Ahaustral margin.
- Air-fluid ratio>2:1.
- **Bird of Prey Sign—smooth tapered narrowing at the point of torsion.**

Blunt Trauma

Gold standard investigation is diagnostic peritoneal lavage (DPL), next best investigation is CT scan abdomen.

Ischaemic Colitis**

- Thumb printing (due to marked mucosal edema)
- **Splenic flexure (watershed zone between superior and inferior mesenteric vessels.**

LIVER/SPLEEN/PANCREAS/GALL BLADDER

Gall Stones**

- 10% of the gall stones are radio opaque while 90% of renal stones are radio opaque.
- Renal/ureteric stones overlap the spine on lateral X-ray
- Mercedes Benz sign—air in the gall stones.
- Investigation of choice **USG**-ECHOGENIC FOCUS WITH POSTERIOR ACOUSTIC SHADOWING**.
- WES sign (wall-echo-shadow sign) in cholelithiasis with chronic cholecystitis, as the gall bladder is contracted and fibrosed only wall of GB, echo and shadow because of stone is seen called as WES sign.
- **Best investigation for Acute Cholecysititis**: Tc 99 HIDA scan.
- Common bile duct stones on cholangiogram classically shows "meniscus appearance".

Biliary Atresia

- Initial investigation is Tc 99 HIDA/DSIDA scan in which there is non-visualiztion of isotope in bowel, confirmatory investigation is **operative cholangiography.**

Pancreatitis**

- For acute pancreatitis investigation of choice is **Contrast Enhanced CT.**
- Best investigation for chronic pancreatitis—ERCP.
- **Chain of lakes** appearance on ERCP in chronic pancreatitis.
- Pancreatitis may lead to complications like pseudocysts, abscess, and vascular complications like portal/splenic vein thrombosis and pseudoaneurysm formation particularly splenic artery.
- Severity on CT is graded by BALTHAZAR STAGING, on CT pancreas appears bulky, ill-defined peripancreatic planes and shows fluid collections.
- *Plain film findings:* colon cut off, sentinel loop, gasless abdomen, duodenal ileus, mottled lucencies. **
- Pancreatic calcification—Chronic alcoholic pancreatitis (most common), hereditary pancreatitis, malnutrition, hyperparathyroidism.

Annular Pancreas

- Double bubble appearance.
- On ERCP—duct of wirsung is seen to encircle the duodenum—DIAGNOSTIC.

Pancreatic Divisum

- Separate drainage of ventral and dorsal pancreatic ducts, more prone to recurrent pancreatitis.

Periampullary Carcinoma

- Frostberg inverted '3' sign.
- Double duct sign.
  Ca head of pancreas shows Antral pad sign.
- Widening of C-loop.

INDIRECT SIGNS OF PANCREATIC MALIGNANCY

Dilation of the pancreatic duct proximal to a pancreatic mass is a common finding. A normal pancreatic duct usually measures less than 2 to 3 mm and has parallel walls and a straight course. When obstructed, it loses its parallel nature, becomes tortuous, and ends or tapers abruptly. The pancreatic duct distends with aging, but it maintains its parallel straight course and can be followed to its entrance into the duodenum. Recognition of a dilated pancreatic duct is an important. Recognition of a dilated pancreatic duct is an important observation, because it can lead to detection of small pancreatic carcinoma.

Bile duct dilation **is commonly seen with lesions in the head of the pancreas. The gall bladder and cystic duct may or may not be dilated. The level of obstruction may be in the head, above the head, or in the porta hepatis, depending on the extent of the lesion or associated lymphadenopathy. Abrupt termination of the dilated bile duct is strongly suggestive of malignancy. Dilation of the common bile duct, pancreatic duct, or both may occasionally be the only ultrasonographic finding. Although the** double-duct sign (combined dilation of the pancreatic and common bile duct) is also seen with chronic pancreatitis, it usually indicates the presence of pancreatic adenocarcinoma.

Hepatic Lesions

Segmental Anatomy Liver (Fig. 2.6)

BISMUTH-CONINAUD NOMENCLATURE—Liver is divided into segments on the basis of hepatic veins and portal vein. It is divided into caudate lobe (segment 1), right lobe (segment 5,6,7,8) and left lobe (segment 2,3,4). The liver is divided into right and left lobe by a plane passing through middle hepatic vein and inferiorly by a line joining gall bladder fossa with inferior vena cava.

Causes of focal hypoechoic lesions in the liver can be: Abscess, cysts (simple or hydatid), hepatoma (can be hypoechoic or hyperechoic), metastasis, lymphoma, acute hematoma.

No debris or septations points towards a simple cystic lesion with no internal contents most likely cause would be simple hepatic cyst.

Haemangioma

- Characteristically shows delayed persistent enhancement on CT with centripetal fill in.
- Best investigation for hepatic haemangioma is Tc 99 RBC SPECT.
- On MRI it shows "light bulb appearance" on T2 WI.

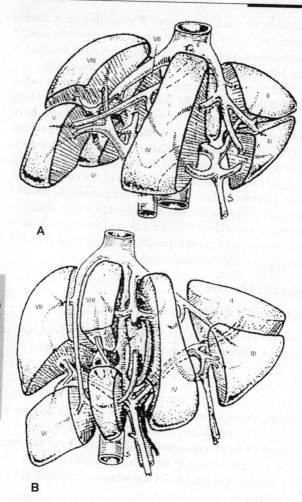

Fig. 2.6: The functional division of the liver and its segments according to Couinaud's nomenclature: (A) as seen in the patient; (B) in the ex-vivo position

Important Points

- Hyper vascular lesions like FNH, adenoma and metastasis from islet cell tumour and RCC etc are best seen in arterial phase CT.
- Metastasis and other focal lesions are best seen in portal venous phase CT, on USG metastasis show characteristic HALO.
- Cholangio Ca is best seen in delayed phase CT due to desmoplastic reaction.

- FNH is rich in Kupffer cells so it's hot or normal on Tc99 colloid scanning.

INTERVENTIONAL RADIOLOGY IN HEPATOCELLULAR CARCINOMA

Percutaneous ethanol injection (PEI)

Transcatheter arterial chemoembolization (TACE) is usually perform in the treatment of large tumors (larger than 3 cm and less than 4 cm in diameter) most frequently performed by intraarterially injecting an infusion of antineoplastic agents mixed with iodized oil (such as Lipiodol).

Radiofrequency ablation (RFA) uses high frequency radio-waves to ablate the tumour.

Intra-arterial iodine-131–lipiodol administration.

High frequency ultrasound (HIFU).

Cryosurgery

As alcohol diffusion is limited in the surrounding cirrhotic liver in HCC it causes damage to the tumour alone with sparing of the normal liver. So, PEI is particularly useful for HCC.

Splenic Trauma

Signs of splenic rupture on plain X-ray are:
- Obliteration of splenic outline (best) **
- Loss of psoas outline.
- Fracture of lower ribs on left side.
- Elevation of left hemidiaphragm.
- Indentation of gastric air bubble.

Adrenal Calcification

- Idiopathic.
- Neoplasm.
- Granuloma.
- Cyst.
- Old hemorrhage.
- Wolman's disease.

Prune Belly Syndrome

- Absent abdominal musculature leading to a wrinkled skin-prune belly.

- Undescended testes.
- Bilateral hydro-ureteronephrosis.

GENITOURINARY SYSTEM

Nephrocalcinosis

Cortical

- Acute cortical necrosis.
- Alports syndrome.
- Graft rejection.
- Hemolytic-uremic syndrome.
- Chronic glomerulonephritis.

Medullary

- Distal renal tubular acidosis.
- Hyperparathyroidism.
- Sarcoidosis and other causes of hypercalcemia.
- Medullary sponge kidney.
- Hyperoxaluria.

Nephrolithiasis

90% of renal calculi are radioopaque.
Radiolucent calculi are:

- Uric acid.
- Xanthine.

Radiopaque calculi are:

- Calcium oxalate and phosphate.
- Struvite.
- Cystine.
- Matrix stones.

  A renal or ureteric calculus overlies the spine on lateral view while a gall stone does not overlie the spine on lateral view.

Acute Ureteric Obstruction

- Increasing dense nephrogram, delayed pyelogram, mild to moderate hydronephrosis.

Chronic Obstruction

- Moderate to gross hydronephrosis, no persistent nephrogram, and poor pyelogram.

Imaging of Ureteric Colic

A plain film of the abdomen and renal ultrasound examination will diagnose most stones. **Spiral CT has emerged as a first-line tool in evaluating flank pain.**

About 90% of calculi are radiopaque (calcium, cystine). Excretory urography is necessary to verify their location within the urinary tract and also affords a qualitative measure of renal function. An acutely obstructed kidney may show only increasing density of the renal shadow without significant radiopaque material in the calices. A nonopaque stone (uric acid) will be seen as a radiolucent defect in the opaque contrast media. Calculi larger than 1 cm cast a specific acoustic shadow on ultrasonography. **Spiral CT has become the study of choice in emergent situations, as the entire urinary tract can be scanned rapidly and without contrast injection. Calculi can be readily identified and distinguished from clot or tumor.** Plain X-ray of the skeletal system may identify Paget's disease, sarcoidosis, or osteoporosis due to prolonged immobilization responsible for hypercalciuria.

Tuberculosis

- Haematogenous route.
- Lobar calcification.
- **Autonephrectomy or Putty kidney****.
- Hiked up renal pelvis, kerrs kink.
- Pipestem or cork screw ureters.
- Small low capacity thick walled bladder or **Thimble Bladder**** bladder calcification is rare in tuberculosis, common in schistosomiasis.
- IVP is the best investigation to detect early tuberculosis (also for early transitional cell Ca which shows a stippled appearance on IVP).
- Feathery appearance of calyces is the earliest sign on IVP.
- Golf hole ureters on cystoscopy.

Cystic Renal Disease

Multicystic Dysplastic Kidney (Potter Type II)

- Kidney is replaced by multiple non-communicating cysts, and is non-functional.
- Usually unilateral.

Polycystic Kidney

- Autosomal dominant or **adult form**—Swiss Cheese Nephrogram, also shows spider leg calyces on IVP.
- Autosomal recessive or **infantile form**—Striated Nephrogram (Potter Type I).
- *Antenatal USG* shows B/L enlarged echogenic kidneys with oligohydramnios.

Simple Cyst

- Characteristic cortical BEAK SIGN on IVP.

CHARACTERISTIC APPEARANCES

Horse Shoe Kidney**

- Flower vase appearance.
- Lower pole calyces point towards each other or shaking hand sign.
- Isthmus may be functional or a fibrous band.
- Prone to trauma, Wilms tumour and obstruction.

Ureterocele

- Adder head appearance on IVP.

Duplex Draining System

- Most common congenital anomaly of the upper urinary tract.
- **Weigert Meyer Law**—upper moiety drains lower in the bladder.
- Upper pole moiety is more prone to obstruction and lower pole more prone to reflux.
- If ureters get fused uretero-ureteric reflux may occur- YO-YO REFLUX.

Medially Placed Ureters on IVP

- Retroperitoneal fibrosis.
- **Other causes:** pelvic lipomatosis, abdominoperineal resection, ureterolysis.

Reflux Nephropathy

- Evaluation with MCU and DMSA scanning.
- Best investigation for demonstrating reflux is-MCU (micturating cystourethrography).

- Grading of VUR.

G-I ureter only.

G-II ureter, pelvis, calyces, no dilatation, normal calyceal fornices.

G-III mild dilatation or tortuosity of ureter and renal pelvis none or minor blunting of fornices.

G-IV moderate dilatation /tortuosity of ureter and moderate dilatation of renal pelvis and calyces complete obliteration of sharp angles of fornices but papillary impressions maintained in calyces.

G-V gross dilatation /tortuosity of ureter; gross dilatation of renal pelvis and calyces; calyces show loss of papillary impressions.

TRAUMA

Renal

- Conservative management usually.
- Traditionally IVP is the investigation of choice not only to look for the damaged kidney but more importantly to look for the **status of the contralateral kidney.**
- Nowadays CT is the preferred modality; shows associated other organ injury also.

Bladder

- Can be intraperitoneal or extraperitoneal.
- On cystography in intraperitoneal rupture contrast will be seen outlining the bowel loops.

TUMOURS

Most common renal tumour in < 6 months of age—**mesoblastic nephroma.**

Wilms Tumour

- Vascular displacement.
- Areas of necrosis.
- Distortion of pelvicalyceal system.
- Pulmonary metastasis.

Mesoblastic Nephroma

Most common renal tumour in less than 6 months of age.

Neuroblastoma

- Vascular encasement.
- Solid appearance on USG.
- Calcification.
- Bone metastasis.
- Secondaries to orbit with proptosis.

Oncocytoma

- Characteristic Spoke Wheel Pattern on angiography (not considered typical according to recent literature).

Angiomyolipoma

- Associated with tuberous sclerois**.
- Fat containing lesion.
- Hamartoma with fat, blood vessels and smooth muscles.

Renal Cell Carcinoma

- Kidney is non-functioning due to vascular invasion.
- *Bony metastasis*—lytic expansile lesions (also in thyroid) **.
- *Robsons Staging:* Adrenal involvement STAGE II not IV; as kidney and adrenal are within the same fascia.

Renal artery stenosis can be divided into two categories: atheromatous and nonatheromatous.

Atheromatous Renal Artery Stenosis: When atheroma affects the renal arteries, it is likely that other arteries will also be involved. It occurs most commonly in men over the age of 50 and may be detected incidentally when patients are being investigated for coronary artery disease or peripheral vascular disease. Atheromatous renal artery stenosis (ARAS) usually affects the proximal third of the renal artery and may involve the origin of the artery, when it is described as being osteal.

Nonatheromatous Renal Artery Stenosis: Fibromuscular dysplasia (FMD) is the most common cause of a nonatheromatous renal artery stenosis and this typically occurs in young women. The most common form of FMD is medial fibroplasia, when there is the typical 'string of beads' on angiography. This is produced by multiple ring-like stenoses separated by segments of dilated artery that can progress to aneurysms. The proximal third of the renal arteries is generally spared and it usually affects the distal mainstem, but may also involve the major branches. The aorta is spared, but other major arteries, particularly the external iliac artery and the carotid arteries, can be involved.

Takayasu's Disease

This tends to affect younger patients, particularly from South East Asia and India.

Other causes: Middle aortic syndrome is a rare condition in which renal artery stenoses are associated with abdominal aortic coarctation and often with visceral artery stenoses. There is also an association between neurofibromatosis and renal artery stenosis, which may be bilateral and may be associated with aortic disease.

Signs of significance of renal artery stenosis on an angiogram is:

    a. A percentage diameter stenosis> 70%.
    b. Presence of collaterals.
    c. A systolic pressure gradient> 20 mm Hg across the lesion.
    d. Post stenotic dilatation of the renal artery.

However, presence of collaterals is the most important sign.

Endovascular Treatment of renal artery stenosis includes: angioplasty and stenting.

NEPHROGRAPHIC PATTERNS

Increasingly Dense Nephrogram

- Acute obstruction.
- Acute hypotension.
- Acute pyelonephritis.
- Multiple myeloma, amyloid.
- Acute glomerulonephritis.
- Renal vein thrombosis.
- Acute papillary necrosis.

Striated Nephrogram

- Medullary sponge kidney.
- Infantile or AR polycystic kidney disease.
- Acute pyelonephritis.
- Acute ureteric obstruction.

'Rim Sign' in Nephrogram

- Severe hydronephrosis of the kidneys.
- Acute complete arterial obstruction.

Role of Radionuclide Imaging

- **Functional imaging** or dynamic renography* -**GFR** – **TC^{99} DTPA****
  MAG3 (better functional agent has tubular extraction however is costly)**
- **Static imaging** or anatomical imaging: **TC^{99} DMSA** – e.g., for evaluation of Scars in reflux nephropathy**
- For **renovascular hypertension** screening use Captopril DTPA scanning, gold standard—renal angiography.

Acute Scrotal Pain

- Scrotal scintigraphy is highly sensitive and specific to diagnose acute torsion.

HEAD AND NECK INCLUDING CENTRAL NERVOUS SYSTEM

Normal Intracranial Calcification

Causes

- Pineal, habenulae.
- Choroids plexus.
- Dura (falx, tentorium; over vault).
- Ligaments (petroclinoid and interclinoid).
- Pacchionian bodies.
- Basal ganglia and dentate nucleus.
- Pituitary.
- Lens.

Basal Ganglia Calcification

Causes

- Idiopathic.
- Pseudohypoparathyroidism.
- Familial.
- Hypoparathyroidism.
- Fahr's syndrome.
- Cockaynes syndrome.

SECTION TWO

- CO, Pb poisoning.
- Toxoplasmosis.

Note: Calcification is periventricular in congenital CMV infection while it is scattered in TOXOPLASMOSIS.

TUMOURS

Raised Intracranial Tension

Earliest Sign

- Adults—dorsum sella erosion.
- Children—sutural diastasis.

Other features—increased convolutional markings-'**copper-beaten appearance**'.

Best investigation for all brain tumours is CE (contrast enhanced) MR study.

Meningioma

Plain Film Signs

- Hyperostosis.
- Calcification.
- Increased vascular markings.
- Pneumosinus dilatans.

Craniopharyngioma

- Midline suprasellar calcification in over 80% childhood cases.

Acoustic Neuroma

Investigation of choice is Gd enhanced MRI especially for intracanalicular lesions.

Lipoma of Corpus Callosum

- Bracket calcification.

Brain Tumors which Spread via CSF

- Germ cell tumors.
- Medulloblastoma.
- CNS lymphoma.
- Ependymoma.
  Neoplasms showing calcification are:
  - Craniopharyngioma—calcification in over 75% of cases.

- Glioma-oligodendroglioma shows calcification in 50% cases, posterior fossa glioma in over 20%.
- *Meningioma—in 10%.*
- **Ependymoma—unusual but if seen dense.**
- Papilloma of choroid plexus—around 25% calcify.
- Pinealoma.
- Chordoma.
- Dermoid, epidermoid and teratoma.
- Hamartoma.
- Lipoma (bracket calcification in lipoma of corpus callosum).

Mnemonic: "Ca2+ COME"

Craniopharyngioma
Astrocytoma, Aneurysm
Choroid plexus papilloma
Oligodendroglioma
Meningioma, Medulloblastoma
Ependymoma.

NEURO-CUTANEOUS SYNDROMES

Neurofibromatosis

Autosomal Dominant

NF-1 / peripheral neurofibromatosis
- Long arm of chromosome 17
- Café-au-lait spots hallmark—in 100% of patients
- Axillary or inguinal freckling
- Presence of neurofibromas
- Osseous lesions like—hypoplastic sphenoid wing, sutural defects, kyphoscoliosis, dural ectasia, meningoceles
- Ocular manifestations like—optic nerve gliomas in 15%, Lisch nodule in iris, buphthalmos, retinal phakomas, plexiform neurofibroma
- Musculo-skeletal lesions like—ribbon ribs, tibial bowing, pseudoarthrosis, focal overgrowth of digit, rib or limb.
  NF-2 or central neurofibromatosis—10% of all cases of NF
- Chromosome 22
- B/L acoustic schwannomas
- Multiple meningiomas
- Non-neoplastic intracranial calcifications (especially choroids plexus).

SECTION TWO

Sturge Weber Syndrome or Encephalotrigeminal Syndrome

- Usually sporadic.
- Capillary or cavernous haemangioma with focal seizure which typically occurs opposite to the side to the lesion.
- **Tram track calcification:** Mainly occipital region
- Associated atrophy
- Ocular –buphthalmos, scleral/choroidal angiomata.

Tuberous Sclerosis

- Autosomal dominant
- Clinical triad of epilepsy, mental retardation and adenoma sebaceum.

CNS Lesions

- Subependymal nodules in brain
- Cortical tubers—Candle drippings, may cause hydro-cephalus
- Retinal phakomas
- Subependymal giant cell astrocytoma at the foramen of monro.

Non-CNS Lesions

- Skin–facial angiofibromas, subungual fibromas, shagreen patch.
- Kidneys—Renal cysts and angiomyolipoma.
- Miscellaneous—Cardiac rhabdomyomas, Honeycomb lung, liver adenomas and leiomyomas, spleen and pancreatic adenomas.

Von Hippel Lindau Syndrome

- Autosomal dominant.
- Gene –chromosome 3p25.

CNS Lesions

- Cerebellar, spinal cord, retinal haemangioblastomas common.

Non CNS lesions

- Cystic lesions of kidneys, pancreas, liver and epididymis.

SECTION TWO

- Pheochromocytomas
- Renal cell carcinoma also common.

CRANIOSYNOSTOSIS

- Craniosynostosis is the premature fusion of the cranial sutures. Craniosynostosis can occur as an isolated defect or as part of a syndrome.
- Synostosis of the sagittal suture produces a long and narrow skull, called scaphocephaly or dolichocephaly. The anteroposterior diameter of the skull is increased, whereas the transverse diameter is decreased.
- Synostosis of the coronal suture can occur bilaterally or unilaterally and is called brachycephaly and plagio-cephaly, respectively. Brachycephaly results in a short, wide skull, with a shortened anteroposterior diameter with a flattened occiput and forehead.
- Synostosis of the metopic suture occurs in utero. It is rare and called trigonocephaly.
- A combined synostosis of the coronal and sagittal sutures results in a severe form termed oxycephaly, which leads to microcephaly.
- The most common syndrome-associated synostoses are Crouzon disease and Chotzen and Apert syndromes, which account for more than two thirds of syndrome-related craniosynostosis.
  1. **Crouzon disease** is inherited as an autosomal domi-nant trait in 75% of patients, whereas the remaining cases are sporadic. The shape varies depending on the order of fusion, but it most commonly results in brachycephaly due to closure of the coronal and basal skull sutures. Associated findings include ocular proptosis, maxillary hypoplasia, parrot-beak nose, and ocular hypertelorism with normal limbs. Hydrocephalus is more common than in the other syndromes. Chronic tonsillar herniation is a common MRI finding that is seen in patients with Crouzon disease.
  2. **Apert syndrome** (acrocephalosyndactyly) is an autosomal dominant disorder characterized by coronal synostosis in conjunction with a malformed and short cranial base. It is associated with extensive syndactyly of the second, third, and fourth fingers **(mitten hands),** broad thumbs with radial deviation,

toe syndactyly **(sock toes),** and visual impairment. Risk of mental retardation is increased; one half of patients have an intelligence quotient lower than 70. Cervical vertebrae fusion, primarily at the C5-C6 vertebrae, occurs in 68% of patients.

3. **Carpenter syndrome** is inherited as a rare autosomal recessive trait and usually results in the kleeblattschädel deformity. Soft tissue syndactyly is always present in the hands and feet. Mental retardation is common.

STROKE

- Ischaemic stroke detected earlier on MRI (esp. DW MRI) diffusion weighted imaging. **
- Haemorrhage detected earlier on NCCT head.

  Acute SAH <48 hours—CT is the investigation of choice

  Chronic SAH > **48 hrs–MRI investigation of choice***

  *Biconvex hyperdense – **extradural hemorrhage**–Arterial (due to rupture of middle meningeal artery)

  *Concavo-convex–**Subdural hemorrhage**–Venous (due to cortical bridging veins rupture). Density of hemorrhage decreases with time and clears from periphery.

  Venous sinus thrombosis—increased density of dural sinuses with lack of normal enhancement—DELTA SIGN.

  Reversal of blood flow in the ipsilateral vertebral artery due to subclavian (proximal) narrowing subclavian steal syndrome.

CHARACTERISTIC APPEARANCES

Large Head in Infancy

- Hydrocephalus.
- Subdural effusion.
- Normal.
- Migrational anomaly.
- Lipidoses.
- Spongy degeneration.
- Alexander's disease.
- Tuberous sclerosis.

Histiocytosis **

- Geographic lytic lesion in skull with beveled edges.
- Button sequestrum.

- Floating teeth.
- Vertebra plana—most common site thoracic spine (other rare d/d of collapse of a single vertebral body—Ewing's tumor, metastasis from a neuroblastoma, benign osteoblastoma or rarely bizarre atypical T.B. focus).
- Honeycomb lung.
- Hand schuller Christian disease triad of exophthalmos, diabetes insipidus and skull lesions.

Basal Exudates on CT

Characteristic of tuberculosis, cryptococcosis (cryptococcosis also shows prominent Virchow robbin spaces). Other features of TB meningitis are—communicating hydrocephalus, infarcts due to tubercular endarteritis.

Myelography

- **Extradural block**- feathered appearance.
- **Intradural extramedullary block**—meniscus sign, with widening of the ipsilateral subarachanoid space.
- **Intramedullary block** widening of the cord, trouser leg appearance.

Cranial USG

- Transfontanelle USG is used in infants.
- Open fontanelles—rationale behind use.
- No radiation.
- Easy/portable.
- Mainly used for diagnosis and follow up of hydrocephalus.

CONGENITAL DISORDERS

Arnold Chiari Malformation *** (Fig. 2.7)

- Type 1 is the mild form with just tonsillar herniation, type 2 has dorsolumbar myelomenigocele and types 3 and 4 have cerebellar hypoplasia and high cervical or occipital encephalocele.

Other Associated Malformations

- Fenestrated falx with interdigitations of cerebral gyri.
- Tectal beaking.
- Lacunar skull.
- Forward bowing of pterous bones and clivus.

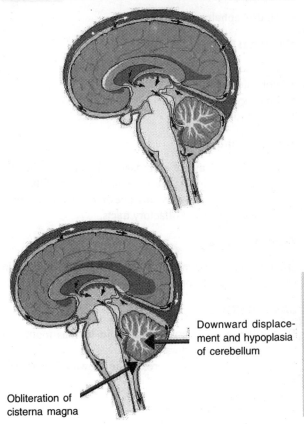

Fig. 2.7: Arnold Chiari Malformation

- Medullary kink.
- Synringohydromyelia.
- Craniovertebral junction anomalies.
- Small posterior fossa.
- Malformed midline cerebellum with extension of vermis through foramen magnum.
- Lemon sign, banana sign.

Dandy Walker Malformation

- Membranous obstruction of foramen of magndie and luschka
- Hypoplastic cerebellum
- Agenesis or hypoplasia of cerebellar vermis
- Posterior fossa cyst
- Expanded posterior fossa

- Hydrocephalus.

Neuronal Migrational Disorders

- Lissencephaly.
- Polymicrogyria.
- Pachygyria.
- Heterotopias.

Holoprosencephaly

- Failure of cleavage of prosencephalon into diencephalons and telencephalon leading to fusion of thalami, monoventricular cavity, absence of falx cerebri, corpus callosum, optic and olfactory tracts.

Schizencephaly

Bilateral clefts extend from ventricles to convexity in operculoinsular region.

JAW LESIONS

Radicular cyst: Related to root of a carious tooth and absorbs local lamina dura.
Dentigirous cyst: Cyst is related to crown of unerupted tooth.

Ameloblastoma

- Mainly in the molar region of the mandible.
- Radiologically—thinning of cortex in bucco-lingual plane, multilocular cystic 'soap bubble' or 'honey-comb' appearance.

Calcifying Epithelial Odontogenic Tumor (PindborgTumor)

The calcifying epithelial odontogenic tumor (CEOT) is a benign infiltrative odontogenic tumor that is one of the most rare. It is most often is found in the mandibular molar/ premolar region, but 33% of the cases are found in the maxilla. It is associated with an unerupted or impacted tooth 50% of the time. It is an infiltrative neoplasm and causes destruction with local expansion. It is less aggressive than ameloblastoma **Radiographic Findings snow-driven appearance.**

Decreased Teeth Enamel

Generalised
- Hyperparathyroidism.
- Cushing's syndrome.
- Osteomalcia.
- Pagets.
- Scleroderma.

Localised
- Leukemia.
- Metastasis.
- Lymphoma.

Pantomography used for jaw lesion and TM joint.

WHITE MATTER DISORDERS

MRI is the most sensitive modality.

Can be classified into demyelinating like multiple sclerosis, central pontime myelinolysisetc and dysmyelinating including leukodystrophies and metabolic disorders.

Multiple Sclerosis

- Shows periventricular plaques especially on T2 weighted MR.
- Dawson's fingers—perivenular areas of demyelination.
  Herpes simplex encephalitis classically involves bilateral temporal lobes and sub frontal regions.

MISCELLANEOUS

Juveline Angiofibroma

- Intracranial extension is best assessed by gadolinium enhanced MRI.
- Classical sign is anterior bowing of the posterior antral wall or "antral bow sign" due to the widening of the pterygo-maxillary fissure.

Laryngeal Malignancy

MRI best assesses cartilage involvement and base of tongue involvement.

Blow Out Fractures Orbit

Herniation of orbital fat and periorbita into maxillary or ethmoid sinuses—tear drop appearance.

Graves Ophthalomopathy

* Enlargement of extraocular muscles with enlargement confined to muscle belly and sparing of tendinous insertions.

Cavernous Haemangiomas

* Most common benign orbital tumours in adults.

OBSTETRICS AND GYNAECOLOGY

OBSTETRICS

Best For Dating
* 1st TRIMESTER US.

Best Parameter in Each Trimester

* 1st – CRL.
* 2nd – BPD.
* 3rd – FL AND HC.
  Where,
  CRL crown rump length
  BPD biparietel diameter
  FL femur length
  HC head circumference.

	TVS	TAS
Gsac	4.5 weeks	5 weeks
Yolk Sac	5 weeks	6-7 weeks
Embryo	6 weeks	6-7 weeks
Ventricles	8.5 weeks	11 weeks
Spine	7-8 weeks	12 weeks
Fetal Heart	5.5 weeks	6.5 weeks

WHERE TVS-Transvaginal sonography, TAS is transabdominal sonography.

IUGR

* Symmetrical-chromosomal

- Asymmetrical –uteroplacental insufficiency; affects trunk>head, earliest parameter to be affected is AC (abdominal circumference).

Earliest Congenital Anomaly That Can Be Detected On USG

Anencephaly: symmetric absence of cranial vault and brain structures above large and prominent orbits, diagnosis is suspected by 12-13 weeks and reliable around 15-16 weeks.

Hydrops Fetalis

Sonographic features of hydrops are:
- Skin thickening more than 5mm, placental enlargement greater than 4 cm, ascites, pleural and pericardial effusion and polyhydramnios.

Signs of Fetal Death

- Roberts's sign: Gas in heart and great vessels-as early as 12 hours.
- Spalding sign overlapping of cranial bones 7 days after
- Hyperflexion of spine.

GYNECOLOGY

Ultrasound Appearance of Normal Endometrium

- Thin echogenic line-early proliferative phase.
- Trilaminar appearance-periovulatory phase.
- Thick echogenic-secretory phase.
- Broken line-menstruating.

Date of Cycle	Phase	Thickness	Appearance
1-4	Menstrual phase	1-4	Thin interrupted central echo
5-14	Proliferative		
	Periovulatory	4-8	Mildly echogenic surrounded by thin hypoechoic band Multilayered with echogenic line of opposing endometrium and echogenic outer rim
15-28	Secretory phase	8-16	Thick,echogenic

Radiological Signs of Ovulation

- Free fluid in pouch of Douglas.
- Collapse of follicle.
- Trilaminar appearance of endometrium.

Ectopic Pregnancy

- No intrauterine gestational sac with ß HCG>1800mIU/ml suggests a diagnosis of ectopic pregnancy.
- Double decidual sac sign a sensitive and specific indicator of intrauterine pregnancy.
- Co existent intra and extra uterine gestations occur in 1/30000 pregnancy.
- **Presence of complex adnexal mass with or without live embryo is the most important sign.**

  Transvaginal ultrasound is useful earliest at 1500-2000 human chorionic gonadotropin(MIU/ml). During normal pregnancy, serum HCG levels double every 2-3 days and are 50-100 mIU/mL at the time of the first missed menstrual period. Peak levels are reached 60-80 days after the last menstrual period (LMP) (30,000 100,000 mIU/mL), and levels then decrease to a plateau of 5,000-10,000 mIU/mL at about 120 days after

  LMP and persist until delivery.

Hydatiform Mole

On USG shows snowstorm appearance.**

Choriocarcinoma

Pulmonary metastases is taken as stage III
Pulmonary metastases appearances are:
- Discrete masses.
- Miliary or snowstorm pattern.
- Pulmonary hypertension or infarction.

Pelvic Malignancy

- MRI is the investigation of choice in staging of pelvic malignancies.

BREAST IMAGING

- Signs of carcinoma on mammography:***

Role to detect DCIS (ductal carcinoma in situ), in screening for breast cancer:

Important Sign of Malignancy

- **CLUSTERED micro calcifications* (more than 5 particles in 1 cm³ of less than 0.5 mm size).**

Other features

- Undefined margins
- Spiculations
- Architectural distortion

  Pop corn pattern of calcification in breast-fibroadenoma

  For **breast implant evaluation** best investigation is MRI***.

SOFT TISSUES

Ear Cartilage Calcification

- Most common—frost bite
- Alkaptonuria
- Cushing syndrome
- Addison's disease
- Relapsing polychondritis.

Parasitic Calcification Causes

- Cysticercus cellulosae
- Loaisis
- Guinea worm
- Armillifer armillatus.

'Magic Angle Effect'

- Signal artefact is seen within tendons, which are oriented 55 degree to the magnetic field. Seen on T1 weighted image not on T2 image.

Section 3

Radiotherapy

DEFINITIONS

Treatment of diseases by means of Roentgen rays or other forms of radioactivity.

Synonyms: Actinotherapy, irradiation, radiation, radiation therapy.

Other forms can be Gamma rays, or particles like electrons, protons, neutrons, positrons, alpha particles.

X-Rays: Electromagnetic radiation of short wavelength approximately 0.01nm to 200 nm produced when high-speed electrons strike solid target (usually anode). These are powerful enough to penetrate most substances except heavy metals (such as lead and gold).

Gamma Rays: Very penetrating rays not appreciably deflected by magnetic or electric field emitted by radioactive substances. The prevailing view is that they are non periodic ether pulses differing from X-ray only in being more penetrating.

Electron: An elementary particle with negative charge.

Proton: Stable particle with positive charge equal to negative charge of electron with mass of about 1 amu. It exhibits a bragg peak.

Neutron: Elementary particle with zero charge and mass about equal to proton i.e. 1 amu. It enters into structure of atomic nucleus.

Positron: An elementary particle with positive charge. Interaction of positron with electron results in annihilation. It is also called as antielectron.

Alpha Particle: A positively charged particle that is nucleus of helium atom emitted from natural or radioactive isotopes has 2p+2n and a charge of + 2.

Sources of Radiation Exposure	
Natural	*Man-made*
1. Cosmic rays	1. Medical and dental: X-rays, Radioisotopes
2. Environmental : 1. Terrestrial 2. Atmospheric	2. Occupational exposure
3. Internal: **Potassium –40** Carbon –14	3. Nuclear : Radioactive fallout
	4. Miscellaneous: Television sets Radioactive dial Watches, Isotope Tagged products Luminous markers

Natural

A. **Cosmic rays**: Originate in outer space and pass through atmosphere
At normal living altitudes exposure 35 mrad/year. At altitudes above 20 Km cosmic radiation becomes important.

B. **Environmental**:
   i. *Terrestrial radiation:* Radioactive elements such as thorium, uranium, radium and an isotope of potassium (K40), exposure-50mrad/year, Highest in Kerala.
   ii. *Atmospheric radiation:* From Radioactive gas as Radon, Thoron, and exposure-2 mrad/year.

C. **Internal Radiation**: These radioactive materials include minute quantities of uranium, thorium and related substances, and isotopes of potassium (K40), strontium (Sr90), and carbon (C14), exposure-25 mrad/year may be upto 70/80.
   Total Natural Radiation Exposure on Average—0.1 rad/ year.

Sources of Natural Radiation

Three series:
* Actinium
* Uranium
* Thorium.

SECTION THREE

Uranium 235 - Actinium Series
0.72% of all natural uranium
704 million years half life
Uranium 238 - Uranium Series.
99.2745% of all natural uranium, 4.7 ppm in common rocks.
4.47 billion years half-life.

Uranium-238	4.47 billion years	alpha, X-rays
Thorium-234	24.1 days	beta, gamma, X-rays
Protactinium-234m	1.17 minutes	beta, gamma
Uranium-234	245,000 years	alpha, X-rays
Thorium-230	77,000 years	alpha, X-rays
Radium-226	1600 years	alpha, gamma
Radon-222	3.83 days	alpha
Polonium-218	3.05 minutes	alpha
Lead-214	26.8 minutes	beta (700 keV), gamma, X-rays
Bismuth-214	19.7 minutes	beta (0.5, 3 MeV), gamma
Polonium-214	164 microseconds	alpha
Lead-210	22.3 years	beta, gamma, X-rays
Bismuth-210	5.01 days	beta
Polonium-210	138 days	alpha
Lead-206	Stable	

Thorium 232 - Thorium Series		
1.6 to 20 ppm in common rocks		
14.1 billion years half life		
Thorium-232	14.1 billion years	alpha, X-rays
Radium-228	5.75 years	beta
Actinium-228	6.13 hours	beta, gamma, X-rays
Thorium-228	1.91 years	alpha, gamma, X-rays
Radium-224	3.66 days	alpha, gamma
Radon-220	55.6 seconds	alpha
Polonium-216	0.15 seconds	alpha
Lead-212	10.64 hours	beta (335 keV), gamma, X-rays
Bismuth-212	60.6 minutes	alpha, beta, gamma, X-rays
Polonium-212	0.305 microseconds	alpha
Thallium-208	3.07 minutes	beta, gamma
Lead-208	Stable	

Other Natural Sources

- Potassium 40
- Rubidium 87
- Carbon 14
- Tritium 3
- Beryllium 7

Man Made Sources

I. X-ray
II. Radioactive fallout:
   Important sources carbon (C14), Iodine (I131), cesium (Cs137) and strontium (Sr90) Cs137 and Sr90 are considered most important because they are liberated in large amounts and remain radioactive for many years.
III. Miscellaneous—TV, watches, etc.

Law of Radioactive Decay

Nuclear decay, being the source of natural radioactivity, is a phenomenon that cannot be stopped by chemical means: A (radioactive) unstable atomic nucleus undergoes disintegration, whatever the chemical nature of the corresponding atom may be. The transformation of a parent nucleus in a daughter nucleus always follows a kinetic law of 1st order, whatever the radioactive nucleus may be and whatever the mode of decay may be.

The velocity of nuclear disintegration (variation of the number of nuclei present with time, $-dN/dt$) is proportional to the number of nuclei present (N). The proportionality constant (k) is called disintegration constant and is characteristic of a radioactive nucleus.

1st order process:
$$-dN/Dt = k.N$$

Where,
   N: number of radionuclei present
   $-dN/dt$: velocity of radioactive decay
   k: disintegration constant.

TYPES OF RADIATION

1. **Electromagnetic Radiation**
   The following are all the same form of energy—they only differ in the amount of energy in the energy packets (photons) that they contain.
   • Radiowaves
   • Microwaves
   • Infrared
   • Visible light
   • Ultraviolet
   • X-Rays and Gamma Rays

Characteristics:
- All have same velocity
- High frequency and smaller wavelength
- Greater power of penetration.
- It has higher energy.

2. **Corpuscular**: It has low penetration power
Examples are alpha particles, beta particles (electrons) and protons.

Type of Radiation	Approximate penetrating ability Air	Tissue	Lead
Alpha Particles	4 cm	0.05 mm	0
Beta Particles	6-300 cm	0.06-4.0 mm	0.005-0.3 mm
Gamma rays	400 metres	50cm	0.3 mm
X-rays	120-240 metres	15-30 cm	0.3 mm
Cosmic rays		Some components very high	

MECHANISM OF ACTION OF RADIATION

- DNA is the primary target for radiation induced cell death.

Ionising radiation generates free radicals and reactive oxygen intermediates that damage local cellular constituents, especially DNA. **DNA double stranded breaks are critical lesion** that results in cell death.

Types and Frequency of Radiation-induced Damage

Type of damage	Number per Gy per cell
DNA double-strand breaks	40
DNA single-strand breaks	1000
DNA–protein crosslinks	150
DNA–DNA crosslinks	30
Base damage	2000
Sugar damage	1500

Radiation-induced Chromosome Aberrations

Chromosome breaks can occur when cells are irradiated. The broken ends of chromosomes can combine with broken ends of different chromosomes. These abnormal combinations are most readily seen during mitosis. Chromosome abnormalities typically occur in cells irradiated in the G1 phase of the cell cycle, before the doubling of genetic material. If cells are irradiated in the G2 phase, chromatid aberrations may result. The frequency of chromosomal aberrations in peripheral circulating lymphocytes correlates with the dose received. The dose can be estimated by comparing the chromosomal changes to in vitro cultures exposed to controlled doses of irradiation. **The minimum dose that can be detected by peripheral lymphocyte analysis is about 0.1 to 0.2 Sv (10 to 20 rem).** Lymphocyte analysis may provide evidence of recent total-body exposure.

Three steps are described for damage:
• Ionization
• Free Radical Generation
• Oxygen Dependent DNA (and other molecules) damage.

Cellular demise associated with DNA breaks may occur within several hours or may become apparent only after cellular division process then termed as MITOTIC CELL DEATH. In either instance, the process of programmed cell death or apoptosis may ensue after radiation induced cell damage in normal or tumor cells.

The tumor suppressor gene p53 is key regulator of apoptosis. In high percentage of tumors, mutation or suppression of p53 gene may affect ability of tumor cells to undergo programmed cell death in response to ionizing radiation. Cells that don't undergo apoptosis may succumb to necrosis, a process whereby cellular membrane integrity is lost before DNA degradation.

Radiation causes cell to get arrested in G2 phase of cell cycle before mitosis (M) phase and hence cells are most vulnerable to radiation at G2M interface.

In contrast maximum resistance to radiation is seen in 's' and late 'G2' phase of cell cycle.

(*Note:* CELL is very sensitive to heat in S phase. Hence heat and radiation may have additive effect in cell damage).

Effect of Mitosis

Law of Bergonie: Radiosensitivity of a cell varies directly with the rate of mitosis and indirectly with degree of differentiation.

In accordance with this law, rapidly proliferating normal tissues such as intestinal mucosa, bone marrow, and skin are particularly susceptible to ionizing radiation and readily show evidence of cytotoxicity. With slowly proliferating tissues, radiation-induced damage may not be apparent until much later or may occur only after stress to the normal tissues.

Effect of Oxygen: Oxygen concentration is also important in determining radiation sensitivity. Oxygen is important for generating and sustaining the free radicals produced by the radiation.

Hypoxic tissues are relatively resistant to effects of radiation.

At a time in a tissue 10-20% cells are in hypoxic phase. It takes two to three times higher radiation dosage to kill anoxic cells as oxygenated ones.

Vascularity: Poorly vascularised tissues in central areas of large tumor masses are likely to exhibit relative insensitivity to radiation.

THE OXYGEN EFFECT

Oxygen is important to the effects of irradiation. Cells that are irradiated in the absence of oxygen are much more resistant to radiation than those irradiated in oxygen. This is due to the oxygen molecules reacting with free radicals to produce chemically unrepairable peroxy radicals ($R^{.} + O_2$? $RO^{.}_2$). Thus, in effect, oxic cells suffer more DNA damage, the degree of sensitisation by oxygen in often quoted as an oxygen enhancement ratio (OER), which is the ratio of doses needed to produce a given biological effect in the presence or absence of oxygen. For most cells and tissues the OER has a value of around 2:5–3.

The decrease in sensitivity only becomes noticeable at partial pressures of oxygen below around 10 mmHg, which means that most well-vascularised normal tissues (partial pressure of oxygen around 40 mmHg) are not affected by the oxygen effect. However, the vascular supply in tumors usually is not adequate to maintain normal oxygenated conditions for all cells. Oxygen diffusion within a tumor is limited to around 200 µm, so that any tumor with a diameter larger than 400 µm will need to develop a vascular system if the center of the tumor is to remain oxic. The importance of angiogenesis factors that stimulate and control vascular growth is therefore apparent and the potential usefulness of anti-angiogenesis treatments is explained. The recognition of the importance of hypoxia in radiotherapy has led to many attempts to circumvent this problem. It has been observed that patients undergoing pelvic irradiation for cervical cancer have a worse prognosis if their pretreatment haemoglobin level is below 12 g/dl so that it is important to make sure that patients are not anaemic when they start radiotherapy. Some clinical trials have demonstrated a benefit in having the patient breath oxygen at upto three times atmospheric pressure (hyperbaric oxygen, HBO) during irradiation. In head and neck cancer, for example local control and survival have been seen to be 20 percentage points higher at 2 years in the HBO group compared with controls. Such trials demonstrate clearly the importance of hypoxia, though HBO has not been widely adopted, largely for technical reasons.

Examples of genes that have a significant influence on the radiosensitivity of mammalian cells

Gene(s)	Proposed function
Ku70, Ku80, DNAPKcs	Attachment of ends of DNA double strand breaks. Non-homologous end rejoining. Initiation of signal path way?
XRCC2, XRCC3, RAD51	Homologous recombination repair
ATM (ataxia telangiectasia mutated)	Signalling presence of DNA damage?
TP53	Signalling presence of DNA damage?
NBS1 (Nijmegen breakage syndrome1)	Non-homologous end rejoining? Homologous recombination repair
DNA ligase IV	Non-homologous end rejoining.

SECTION THREE

Occupational Cancers

Occupation	Site of tumor	Agent
Dye manufactures; rubber workers	Bladder	Aromatic amines
Copper and cobalt smelters; pesticide manufacture	Skin, lung	Arsenic
Manufacture of chromates from chrome ore	Lung	Chromium
Asbestos miners; asbestos textile manufacturers;	Lung, pleura, peritoneum,	Asbestos

Contd.

Contd.

insulation and shipyard workers	larynx	
Workers with glues and varnishes	Marrow, e.g. erythroleukaemia	Benzene
Uranium and other miners; luminisers; radiologists; radiographers	Lung, bone, bone marrow	Ionising radiation
Nickel refiners	Nasal sinuses, lung	Nickel
Hardwood furniture manufacturers	Nasal sinuses	Agent unknown
Leather workers	Nasal sinuses	Agent unknown
Coal gas manufacturers; asphalters; roofers; aluminium refiners; workers exposed to tars and oils	Skin, scrotum, lung	Polycyclic hydrocarbons (soot, tar and oil)
Seamen; farmers	Skin	Ultraviolet light
PVC manufacturers	Liver (angiosarcoma)	Vinyl chloride

Examples of Radiation-Induced Cancers	
Types of Exposure	*Types of Cancer Observed*
Neck irradiation during infancy for benign conditions	Thyroid carcinoma
Radiation therapy for other malignant tumors	Thyroid carcinoma
	Breast cancer
	Gastric cancer
	Melanoma
	Lung cancer
	Sarcomas in the field
Cranial irradiation	Central nervous system tumors
Breast irradiation for postpartum mastitis	Breast cancer
Brush-licking by radium dial painters	Bone sarcomas
Uranium mining	Lung cancer
In utero exposure	Leukemia

RADIATION UNITS

Rad - unit of "absorbed dose" - energy absorbed per unit mass of tissue

Rem - unit of "equivalent dose"

Equivalent dose = absorbed dose × radiation weighing factor (wR)

wR takes into account that ionizing radiation other than X-rays and gamma-rays can be more damaging to the body for the same amount of absorbed dose.

X-rays and gamma-rays are assigned a radiation weighing factor (wR) of one.
(These other types of ionizing radiation come from radio-active materials, particle accelerators, fission, and fusion, so we don't have to worry about them here. For your infor-mation, though, electrons or beta particles from radioactive decay also have a weighing factor of one, while alpha particles are assigned a weighing factor of 20).

For X-rays (and for gamma-rays): 1 rad = 1 rem, always

New Units (SI units):

Gray (Gy) - unit of "absorbed dose"

Sievert (Sv) - unit of "equivalent dose"

1 Gy = 100 rad   1 Sv = 100 rem.

Unit	Quantity Measured	Definition
Roentgen (R)	Exposure	Amount of X-rays or gamma rays that produces a specific amount of ionization in a given volume of air
Rad	Dose	100 ergs deposited per gram of tissue
Gray (Gy)	Dose	SI unit of dose; equals 100 rad
Rem	Dose equivalence	Unit that reflects the biologic response. It is used to compare various types of radiation
Sievert (Sv)	Dose equivalence	SI unit of dose equivalence; equals 100 rem

For X-rays: 1 Gy = 1 Sv.

SECTION THREE

Effective Dose

The concept of effective dose takes into account the risk to the person exposed to radiation that is not uniform over the entire body.

Different organs have different sensitivities to radiation: This is expressed by the tissue-weighing factor: wT

Tissue Weighing Factors:

Gonads 0.20

Bone Marrow; Colon; Lung; Stomach; 0.12

Bladder; Breast; Liver; Esophagus; Thyroid; Remain-der; 0.05

Bone Surface, Skin 0.01.

PRINCIPLES OF CANCER MANAGEMENT

Surgery alone–the treatment of choice

- Lower oesophagus, stomach, colon, pancreas, kidney
- Thyroid
- Melanoma
- Hepatocellular carcinoma
- Keratoacanthoma.

Radiotherapy—the treatment of choice
- Oral cavity, lip, tongue, cheek
- Nasopharynx
- Oropharynx
- Hypopharynx
- Nasal cavity
- Larynx
- Skin cancer (except melanoma)
- Cervix
- Bladder (except T1)
- Testis–seminoma
- Hodgkin's disease (early)
- Non–Hodgkin lymphoma (early)
- Medulloblastoma (following surgical debulking)
- Astrocytomas (grades 3 and 4)
- Retinoblastoma.

Cytotoxic therapy–the treatment of choice
- Acute and chronic leukaemias
- Hodgkin's disease (advanced)
- Non–Hodgkin lymphoma (advanced)
- Testicular teratoma
- Choriocarcinoma
- Small cell lung cancer
- Rhabdomyosarcoma
- Neuroblastoma.

Radiosensitivity of Different Tumours

Highly sensitive
- Lymphoma
- Seminoma
- Myeloma
- Ewing's sarcoma
- Wilms' tumor.

Moderately sensitive
- Small cell lung cancer
- Breast cancer
- Basal cell carcinoma
- Medulloblastoma
- Teratoma
- Ovarian cancer.

Relatively resistant
- Squamous cell carcinoma of lung
- Hypernephroma
- Rectal carcinoma
- Bladder carcinoma
- Soft tissue sarcoma
- Soft tissue sarcoma
- Cervical cancer.

Highly resistant
- Melanoma
- Osteosarcoma
- Pancreatic carcinoma.

Chemosensitivity of Different Tumors

Highly sensitive (which may be cured by chemotherapy)
- Teratoma of testis Hodgkin's disease
- High–grade non-Hodgkin lymphoma Wilms' tumor
- Embryonal rhabdomyosarcoma
- Choriocarcinoma
- Acute lymphoblastic leukaemia in children
- Ewing's sarcoma.

Moderately sensitive (in which chemotherapy may sometimes contribute to cure and often palliates)
- Small cell carcinoma of lung
- Breast carcinoma
- Low-grade non-Hodgkin lymphoma
- Acute myeloid leukaemia
- Ovarian cancer
- Myeloma.

Relatively insensitive (in which chemotherapy may sometimes produce palliation)
- Gastric carcinoma
- Bladder carcinoma
- Squamous carcinoma of head and neck

- Soft tissue sarcoma
- Cervical carcinoma.

Resistant tumors
- Melanoma
- Squamous carcinoma of lung
- Large bowel cancer.

Note
- Most radiosensitive tissue of body—Bone Marrow.
- Least radiosensitive tissue of body—Nervous tissue/ Brain.
- Most radiosensitive blood cell—Lymphocyte.
- Least radiosensitive blood cell—Platelet.
- Most common organ to be affected by radiation—Skin (erythema earliest change).
- Most radioresistant organ—Vagina.
- Most common mucosa to be affected by radiation- Intestinal mucosa.

METHODS OF RADIOTHERAPY

- Teletherapy.
- Brachytherapy.

TELETHERAPY

Definition: Treatment in which the radiation source is at a distance from the body. Linear accelerators and cobalt machines are used in teletherapy.

Also called external beam therapy.

It is a form of radiation therapy with placement of radioactive source at a distance from the patient (external therapy). With external therapy the source of radiation is placed at a distance 5-10 times greater than the depth of tumor to be irradiated I order to achieve uniform distribution of radiation to the tumor and thereby avoid large dose variation attributable to inverse square law. The distance is called source to skin distance (SSD).

Linear accelerators or Co-60 machines are used commonly for external beam radiation therapy.

Three main types of radiation that are used in radiation therapy-gamma rays, X-rays and electron beams. They are used generally for the same reason and that is to give a dose of radiation to a target in the body. Electron beam therapy is the choice for skin and shallow targets while gamma rays and X-rays will allow for the radiation dose to be given to targets that are deeper in the body.

For gamma radiation we typically use the radioactive material cobalt-60, which is abbreviated as Co-60. It is used because it emits high-energy gamma rays as it decays. Co-60 has a half-life of 5.27 years.

But remember that Co-60 is constantly decaying and that means that it has to be replaced every so often. That is both an inconvenience and a cost to the clinic that uses the machine. Partly for this reason Co-60 teletherapy is being replaced by another machine that uses X-rays to deliver that same dose of radiation, and X-rays are produced by equipment that doesn't rely on a material that has a half-life. These machines are known as linear accelerators (linacs) and have been around for a very long time in many different configurations. In the past few years, however, they have become highly refined in medical applications. In very simple terms, they work by accelerating electrons down a tube that will then either emit them as high energy electrons or X-rays. Making X-rays requires an intermediate step wherein the electrons are aimed to hit a tungsten target. When the electrons hit the tungsten target, they are diverted from their path and are forced to turn and slow down. This causes energy to be given off in the form of an X-ray.

External beam therapy can be broadly divided into kilovoltage therapy and megavoltage therapy depending on the beam quality and their use. Kilovoltage range is further divided into three subcategories.

Kilovoltage Therapy

1. **Contact therapy**

   A contact therapy machine operates at potentials of 40 to 50 kV and facilitates irradiation of accessible lesions at very short source (focal spot) to surface distances (SSD).

2. **Superficial therapy**

   The term superficial therapy applies to treatment with X-rays produced at an energy ranging from **50 to 150 kV**. Varying thicknesses of filters (usually 1 to 6 mm of Al) are used to produce beams of different qualities expressed in terms of half value layer (HVL). The HVL is defined as that thickness of material which reduced the

SECTION THREE

intensity of narrow X-ray beam to half its original
intensity.

3. **Orthovoltage or deep therapy**

The term orthovoltage therapy or deep therapy is used
to describe treatment with X-rays ranging from 150 to
500 kV. Most orthovoltage equipment are operated at
200 to 300 kV.

Supervoltage Therapy

X-ray therapy in the range of 500 to 1000 kV has been
designated as **high voltage therapy or supervoltage
therapy**.

Megavoltage Therapy

X–ray beams of energy 1 MV or greater can be classified
as megavoltage beams. Although the term strictly applies
to the X-ray beams, the gamma-ray beams produced by
radionuclides are also commonly included in this category
if their energy is 1 MeV or greater. Examples of clinical
megavoltage machines are accelerator, betatron, microtron
and the telecobalt units.

Radiation Therapy Simulators

A treatment simulator is an apparatus that uses a diagnostic
X-ray tube but duplicates a radiation treatment unit in terms
of its geometrical, mechanical, and optical properties.[27] The
main function of a simulator is to display the treatment
fields so that the target volume may be accurately
encompassed without delivering excessive irradiation to
surrounding normal tissues.

ROLE OF GATING

Minimizing the planning target volume (PTV) margin and
reproducing its position during treatment as well as between
treatments are important tasks in external beam radio–
therapy. Tumour movement occurs not only as a result of
set-up errors but also from respiration and interferes with
optimized treatment planning. The range of respiratory
motion has been reported to be up to 3.8 cm. Owing to
respiratory movement during irradiation, considerable
margins have to be added around the treatment sites in
thoracic and abdominal regions. Moreover, for moving

organs, especially in intensity-modulated radiotherapy (IMRT), large discrepancies between the intended and delivered planning target volume can be generated, even if there are adequate margins.

<u>Patient respiration during radiotherapy can cause significant motion of the tumour volume, which can be mitigated by gating the accelerator beam to patient respiration.</u>

BRACHYTHERAPY

A type of radiation therapy is which radioactive materials are placed in direct contact with the tissue being treated. Broadly it is of two types—interstitial or intracavitary.

BI   Interstitial
BC   Intra-cavity
BT   Not otherwise specified
US   Unsealed source.

In intracavitary treatment, containers that hold radioactive sources are put into the body cavities that are in or near the tumor (e.g. intrauterine, vagina). In interstitial treatment, radioactive sources are placed directly into the tumor (e.g., in form of needles). These radioactive sources may stay in the patient permanently. Sometimes, the radioactive sources are removed from the patient after several days.

This technique is particularly useful in treating cancers of the cervix, uterus, vagina and certain head and neck cancers. It can also be used to treat breast, brain, skin, esophageal, soft tissue, lung, bladder and prostate cancer.

Sometimes brachytherapy is done in conjunction with external beam therapy. The external beam radiation destroys cancerous cells in a large area surrounding the tumor. Brachytherapy delivers a boost, or higher dose of radiation, to help destroy the main mass of tumor cells.

If a PATIENT has two unrelated diseases both of which require radiotherapy, each course of treatment should be recorded as a primary course. Similarly if a PATIENT has two primary lesions of the same disease, e.g. two rodent ulcers, the treatment of these comprises two primary courses, unless the lesions are in such close proximity that they are to be treated together. If during a course of treatment, a PATIENT starts a further course, the second course should be separately identified.

Brachytherapy sources

Radionuclide	Radiation emitted	Energy	Half-life	Form
Radium–226	Gamma rays	1 MeV	1620 years	Needles, tubes
Caesium–137	Gamma rays	0.66 MeV	30 years	Tubes, needles, pellets
Cobalt–60	Gamma rays	1.25 MeV	5.26 years	Rods
Iridium–192	Gamma rays	0.4 MeV	74 days	Wires
Gold–198	Gamma rays	0.41 MeV	2.7 days	Seeds
Strontium–90	Beta rays	2.27 MeV max	28.1 years	Plaques
Yttrium–90	Beta rays	2.27 MeV max	64 hours	Rods

Radionuclides suitable for unsealed use

Radionuclide	Form in which used	Half-life	Radiation emitted	Method of administration
Iodine–131	Sodium iodide solution	8 days	Beta rays Gamma rays	Oral
Phosphorus–32	Sodium ortho-phosphate solution	14.3 days	Beta rays	Intravenous injection
Yttrium–90	Colloidal liquid	64 hours	Beta rays	Intracavitary injection

Dose rates in brachytherapy

Low dose rate	0.4–2.0 Gy h^{-1}	2 fractions
Medium dose rate	2.0–12 Gy h^{-1}	2 fractions
High dose rate	12–60 Gy h^{-1}	> 6 fractions

Note

The use of **RADIUM–226** ($T_{1/2}$=1640 years) to produce gamma radiation effects in limited volumes of tissue is one of the oldest established practices of radiotherapy. Radium–226 is an alpha emitter but within its decay scheme are radium B (lead–214) and radium C (bismuth–214) emitting gamma rays with energies in the range from 0.2–2.4 MeV; the higher energy photons in the spectrum make radiation protection difficult and the inert gas, radon–222, is a constant additional hazard.

Brachytherapy (implants) can be either temporary or permanent. Temporary implants, as the name implies, only leave the sources in for a short period of time and then they are removed. Temporary implants can be either high dose rate (the sources are left in for a matter of minutes) or medium dose rate (the sources are left in for a matter of days). Permanent implants are placed forever. These implants are low dose rate. Two radioisotopes are used in permanent prostate brachytherapy: Iodine-125 (or ^{125}I) and Palladium-103 (or ^{103}Pd).

Gold seeds are used in treatment of malignant ascites.

Therapeutic Ratio

The ratio of the maximally tolerated dose of a drug to the minimal curative or effective dose; LD50 divided by ED50. i.e. in simple language it is balance between therapeutic effect and damage caused as all cells exposed to radiation undergo some damage. It is percentage of patients cured divided by the cost of the treatment in terms of side-effects. The fewer the side-effects without compromising the chance of cure, the better the therapeutic ratio.

Therapeutic Ratio should be major consideration in deciding radiotherapy and can be improved by *oxygenation, radiosensitisers and hyperfractionation.*

Technical Factors in Radiotherapy

In any radiation treatment the clinician has to define the following parameters:

1. Tumor volume
2. Target volume
3. Treatment volume
4. Radiation energy and quality
5. Number of fields
6. Arrangement of fields
7. Use of wedges, tissue compensators or bolus
8. Dose
9. Total number and frequency of fractions
10. Overall treatment time.

Dose Fractionation and Overall Treatment Time

It is essential to specify dose, energy, number of fractions and overall treatment time together since each has an effect on the biological response. Stating a dose without specifying its energy, fractionation and overall treatment time is meaningless.

Dose in Radical and Palliative Radiotherapy

Radical: In radical radiotherapy the choice of dose and fractionation regime will depend on the radiosensitivity of the tumor, the size of the treatment volume, the proximity of dose-limiting critical structures and the quality of radiation used.

Relatively radiosensitive tumors such as testicular seminoma can be controlled by total doses of 30 Gy at megavoltage fractionated over 4 weeks. Higher doses of the order of 50–55 Gy are needed to control most squamous carcinomas of the head and neck.

The maximum tolerated dose of radical radiotherapy to different volumes of tissue varies in different parts of the body. For example, field sizes in excess of 60 cm^2 for head and neck cancer rarely tolerate more than 50 Gy in 20 daily fractions over 4 weeks. Similarly, the tolerance of the small bowel limits the dose to the whole pelvis in cervical/ endometrial cancer to 45 Gy fractionated over the same period.

The presence of critical structures such as the brainstem and spinal cord may limit the dose that can be delivered to tumors, for example of the head and neck, lung and oesophagus. This problem can be obviated in treating nodal areas overlying the cord in the head and neck by the use of electrons of limited penetration. The appropriate energy can be chosen to ensure that the cord is not overdosed.

The relative biological effectiveness (RBE) of the quality of irradiation chosen will influence the choice of dose. Fast neutrons have a higher RBE than photons. The RBE of neutrons varies in different tissues and increases as the dose per fraction falls. The radical doses of neutrons equivalent to photons are therefore much lower.

Homogeneity of dose distribution across the target volume is important to achieve maximum tumor kill. Areas of underdosage may give rise to local recurrence and overdosage to morbidity. For this reason the variation in dose across the target volume should not vary by more than ±5% of the intended dose.

Palliative. Homogeneity of dose distribution is much less important than in radical radiotherapy. Thus simple treatment techniques by single or parallel—opposed fields will suffice for most purposes. Since dose homogeneity is not essential, computerised planning and the use of wedges to improve the dose distribution are not needed. Treatment volumes should be more generous than for radical radiotherapy since the doses delivered should be well below normal tissue tolerance.

Palliative Radiotherapy

Palliative radiotherapy is aimed at relieving local symptoms of advanced disease. The following criteria should be applied to achieve good palliation:
1. Prompt relief of symptoms
2. Minimal upset from treatment
3. Simple treatment technique
4. Limited number of fractions.

Assessment

Patients with advanced disease may have a life expectancy ranging from a few days to many months. A judgment has to be made as to whether the patient is likely to benefit within his or her expected life span. In most cases benefit from palliative radiotherapy is seen during or within a few days of treatment. Where life expectancy is only a few days, every effort should be made to control the patient's symptoms at home by medical means without recourse to radiotherapy.

Palliative radiotherapy should relieve symptoms with minimal side-effects. The amount of upset varies with site, dose and fractionation.

Site: Sites which tolerate palliative radiotherapy poorly are the upper abdomen (sensitivity of the stomach and duodenum), oral cavity (soreness and dysphagia) and perineum (painful skin and vaginal reaction).

Single fractions of 8 Gy to the lower thoracic and upper lumbar spine are likely to cause vomiting since some of the duodenum will be incorporated in the field. Fractionated treatment is better tolerated. Palliative radiotherapy is of value at a wide range of tumor sites. Here are a few examples.
- Relief of haemoptysis, cough, dyspnoea and mediastinal obstruction in lung cancer.
- Control of bleeding in advanced bladder, rectal and cervical cancer.
- Relief of pain from bone metastases.
- Relief of symptoms of raised intracranial pressure due to brain metastases.
- Healing of ulcerating breast tumors.

Dose and Fractionation

Relatively low doses are adequate to relieve most symptoms. Single fractions of 8 Gy using orthovoltage, cobalt-

60 or megavoltage are suitable for ribs, upper thoracic spine, and long bones. Fractionated doses, e.g. 20 Gy in four daily fractions or 30 Gy in 10 fractions are suggested for bony metastases in the cervical, lower thoracic and upper lumbar spine and for malignant spinal cord compression.

Technique

The treatment setup should be as simple as possible, with single or parallel-opposed fields to limit the duration of each treatment.

FRACTIONATION

Fractionation refers to the division of the total dose into a number of separate fractions, conventionally given on a daily basis, usually 5 days a week (Monday to Friday).

In assessing the value of any fractionation regime, whether for cure or palliation, the effects on both the tumor and the normal tissues have to be considered together. Normal tissue tolerance is dose limiting at many sites in radical radiotherapy (e.g. the spinal cord in head and neck irradiation). At high dose a small increase in cure may be at the expense of substantially greater morbidity. Similarly, high dose per fraction is poorly tolerated with even palliative doses at sensitive sites.

According to the Law of Bergonie and Tribondeau (1904): Radiosensitivity increases with the amount of proliferative activity within tissues at the time of radiation. This is now thought not to be the case. The proliferative state of cells at the time of radiation exposure is not critical. However, for radiation to have an acute effect, cells need to be in a proliferative state at or within a short time of exposure. Anaplastic (or poorly differentiated) tumors have a higher proportion of their cell population in mitosis at any given time than do well-differentiated tumors. It follows that anaplastic growths are more likely to be more radio-sensitive. A single dose of 20 Gy may suffice to cure a small basal cell carcinoma of the skin, but if given in five daily fractions (5×4 Gy) it would be insufficient. To achieve a comparable result would require 5×6 Gy (30 Gy). If we took 2 weeks (10 treatment sessions), the dose would be 10×4.5 Gy (45 Gy). As a general rule, the longer the overall treatment time, the higher the total dose required.

Number of Fractions Per Day

1. **Conventional fractionation:** Daily treatments from Monday to Friday with a gap at weekends remain standard for most radical treatments. However, there is wide variation in the overall treatment time. This varies from 15–16 fractions in 3 weeks in Manchester, with a fraction size of 3.3–3.6 Gy, to 35–40 fractions over 7–8 weeks in the USA, with fraction sizes of 1.8–2.0 Gy.

2. **Hyperfractionation (accelerated fractionation):** Instead of treating once a day, the number of daily fractions can be increased, in practice rarely to more than three. This approach has been explored in tumors where conventionally fractionated radiotherapy has often failed to cure tumors (e.g. cerebral gliomas and advanced lung and head and neck cancer). The rationale for giving more than one fraction per day is based on the 5 Rs of radiobiology.

    a. **Dose per fraction:** There is experimental evidence that as the dose per fraction decreases, so too does the oxygen enhancement ratio (p. 290). Theoretically, with multiple small daily fractions the importance of hypoxia as a cause of radio-resistance in tumors should be less marked compared with normal tissues.

    b. **Morbidity:** In general, accelerated or hyperfractionated treatments are associated with more severe acute reactions. As stated above, acute reactions are determined by the rate of accumulation of dose. Unless mall field sizes are used, the mucous membranes of the head and neck will not tolerate fraction sizes of 2 Gy or more given three times a day or more than 55 Gy in 2 weeks.

    Late reactions are influenced by fraction size and the interval between fractions. Late reactions generally worse when the interval return fractions is less than 4.5 hours.

3. **Hypofractionation:** Hypofractionation refers to the practice of giving less than the conventional five daily fractions per week. This approach is illogical for treating most tumor sites since long gaps between fractions may allow tumor repopulation. In a trial comparing three fractions (hypofractionated) versus five fractions (conventional fractionation) per week in laryngeal cancer, there was a tendency for a higher local recurrence

rate in the patients treated with three fractions a week. Hypofractionation is more logical in treating tumors with a higher capacity for repair, e.g. melanomas and soft tissue sarcomas, and in palliative radiotherapy. A limited number of large fractions may take advantage of the higher fractionation sensitivity of such tumors compared with normal tissues. In palliative radiotherapy single fractions of 4–15 Gy for bone metastases are in general as effective as multiple fractions to total doses of 20–40 Gy. As good and prompt pain relief can be achieved by a single fraction of 8 Gy as by 30 Gy in 10 daily fractions. Two fractions of 8.5 Gy given a week apart are as effective in relieving the symptoms of non-small cell lung cancer as 30 Gy in 10 daily fractions.

THE 5 RS OF FRACTIONATED RADIOTHERAPY

The efficacy of fractionated radiotherapy is clearly determined by the physical and technical aspects of radiation delivery and the biological consequences to the tumor and normal tissue. Building on the seminal suggestion of Withers, it is now recognised that there are five factors that are highly influential in dictating the biological response of the tumor. These are the 5 Rs of Radiotherapy. Two of these, recovery and repopulation, lead to a decrease in response when treatment is prolonged, while two, reassortment and reoxygenation, are beneficial in a fractionated regime. The fifth, radiosensitivity, is the baseline on which the other modifications work.

Radioprotectives	Radiosensitizers
Zinc oxide	Oxygen
Pentoxiphylline	Cisplatin
Etramustine	5-Fluorouracil
Amifostine	Gemcitbine
Chlorhexidine (for stomatitis)	cytochlor
Potassium iodide (for	
thyroid against radioiodine)	Sr2508(Etanidazole)
Melatonin (protective for	Nitroimidazoles—Metronida-
skin mitotic cells against	zole, misinidazole, pimo-
chromosomal damage	nidazol
Antioxidants (vit C,E,A0)	

Intensity-modulated radiation therapy (IMRT) is an advanced mode of high-precision radiotherapy that utilizes computer-controlled x-ray accelerators to deliver precise radiation doses to a malignant tumor or specific areas within the tumor. <u>The radiation dose is designed to conform to the three-dimensional (3-D) shape of the tumor by modulating—or controlling—the intensity of the radiation beam to focus a higher radiation dose to the tumor while minimizing radiation exposure to surrounding normal tissues.</u> Treatment is carefully planned by using 3-D computed tomography (CT) images of the patient in conjunction with computerized dose calculations to determine the dose intensity pattern that will best conform to the tumor shape. Typically, combinations of several intensity-modulated fields coming from different beam directions produce a custom tailored radiation dose that maximizes tumor dose while also protecting adjacent normal tissues.

Because the ratio of normal tissue dose to tumor dose is reduced to a minimum with the IMRT approach, higher and more effective radiation doses can safely be delivered to tumors with fewer side-effects compared with conventional radiotherapy techniques. IMRT also has the potential to reduce treatment toxicity, even when doses are not increased.

<u>Currently, IMRT is being used to treat cancers of the *prostate, head and neck, breast,* thyroid and *lung,* as well as in gynecologic, liver and brain tumors and lymphomas and sarcomas</u>. IMRT is also beneficial for treating pediatric malignancies.

However for lung cancer—There has been much interest in developing techniques for intensity-modulated treatment of lung cancers. <u>There are several technical reasons to delay the widespread use of IMRT for lung cancer at this time</u>. First is the issue of tumor motion. IMRT is not appropriate for mobile targets. Second, there is still some uncertainty about the algorithms used to calculate beamlet doses in very inhomogeneous structures. Third, IMRT achieves highly conformal high-dose regions by increasing volumes that receive relatively low doses. This may be a significant problem because the lung is so sensitive to radiation.

Systemic radionuclides for treatment of bone metastases

Radionuclide	Half-Life	Emission	Energy (MeV)	Status
Phosphorus 32 (32P)	14.2 days	Beta	1.71	Approved
Strontium 89 (89Sr)	50.6 days	Beta	1.492	Approved
Samarium 153 (153Sm)	46.3 hours	46.3 hours	0.81	Approved
Gamma			0.10	
Rhenium 186 (186Re)	90.6 hours	Beta	1.071	Investigational
		Gamma	0.137	
Rhenium 188 (188Re)	16.7 hours	Beta	2.116	Investigational

EFFECTS OF RADIATION

Adverse Effects

I. Stochastic (probabilistic)
II. Non stochastic (deterministic).

Stochastic Effects

These may occur at low radiation dose (though the lower the dose the lower the chance of detrimental effect) and are always delayed.

Stochastic Effects ("Chance Effects")

Stochastic effects occur when cells are not killed, but mutated in some way, such that they either multiply out of control, causing cancer, or they cause hereditary disease which is passed on to any children conceived thereafter.

It is assumed that any dose of radiation could potentially cause stochastic effects, as one single X-ray photon could turn one cell into a cancer cell. The bigger the dose, the more likely the effect will occur. The lower the dose, the less likely. However, it must be mentioned they have no threshold and severity of disease does not vary with dose. Are always delayed.

Non Stochastic (Deterministic)

Deterministic Effects ("threshold effects")
Deterministic effects are where so many cells are killed in an organ that some physical symptoms occur.

Below a certain radiation dose (threshold) too few cells are damaged to cause any real harm (millions of cells die and are replaced in the body every day). Above the threshold dose, the bigger the dose, the more cells are killed, so the worse the effect. Deterministic effects generally occur only at rather high radiation doses (greater than 100 rem) and may be acute or delayed. Deterministic: Cataracts, Skin Erythema & Burns, Acute Radiation Sickness & Death.

Cataracts

- Only occur with X-ray doses greater than 2 Sv (200 rem) for a single exposure.
  The threshold dose for inducing cataracts with multiple X-ray exposures over a period of weeks is more than 5 Sv (500 rem).

Skin Erythema and Burns

- The threshold dose for X-ray exposure from a single examination is about 2 Sv (200 rem). Again, if the exposure is protracted over a period of time—days or weeks – the threshold dose is much higher (Note: Earliest skin change is erythema, layer most commonly affected Stratum basalis.
  Sebaceous gland function does not recover after radiotherapy.
  Pinna and Axilla are common sites of Radionecrosis e.g. for skin doses.

Deterministic effect	Threshold single dose
Transient erythema ("sunburn")***	2 Gy
Temporary epilation (hair loss to area irradiated)	3 Gy
Main erythema	6 Gy
Permanent epilation	7 Gy
Dermal necrosis	18 Gy
Secondary ulceration	20 Gy

Note:
- GIT: Earliest part involved Small bowel mucosa Earliest symptom—Diarrhoea.
- Head and Neck: Oropharyngeal mucositis and xerostomia.

A few dose effect levels

Lethal Whole Body	500 rem (5 Sv)
Acute Dose:	
Minimum Acute Whole	100 rem (1 Sv)
Body Symptomatic Dose:	
Dose below which we have	10 rem (0.1 Sv)
little direct evidence of harm:	
Background Radiation:	0.3 rem or 300 mrem per year (3 mSv per year).

Doses to irradiated tissues	
CT	1 to 5 rem (1000 to 5,000 mrem)
Mammogram	150 to 300 mrem (0.15 to 0.3 rem)
Abdominal X-ray	50 to 500 mrem (0.05 to 0.5 rem)
Chest X-ray	5 to 10 mrem (0.005 to 0.01)

The effective dose from a chest X-ray is less than that from a cross country airline flight.

The average equivalent dose to the bronchial epithelium of a smoker is about 16 rem per year.

Some long interventional procedures can produce skin doses in excess of 200 rem (2 Sv) which can produce skin damage.

ACUTE TOTAL-BODY IRRADIATION

The data regarding the acute effects of total-body irradiation on humans come primarily from Japanese survivors of the atomic bomb, Marshallese exposed to radioactive fallout in 1954, and persons exposed to radiation from the Chernobyl nuclear accident. Early symptoms of acute total-body irradiation, known as the prodromal radiation syndrome, last for a limited time. Clinical manifestations depend on the total-body dose. **At doses >100 Gy, death usually occurs 24 to 48 h later from neurologic and cardiovascular failure. This is known as the cerebrovascular syndrome.** Because cerebrovascular damage causes death very quickly, the failures of other systems do not have time to develop.

At doses between 5 and 12 Gy, death may occur in a matter of days as a result of the gastrointestinal syndrome. The symptoms during this period may include nausea, vomiting, and prolonged diarrhea for several days leading to dehydration, sepsis, and death. A total-body dose >10

Gy is uniformly fatal unless supportive therapy (fluid, electrolytes, blood products, and antibiotics) is given. The process of intestinal denudation depends on the dose and may take between 3 and 120 days. Death from intestinal denudation usually occurs before the full effects of radiation on the blood-forming elements are seen.

At total-body doses between 2 and 8 Gy, death may occur 2 to 4 weeks after exposure from bone marrow failure, the hematopoietic syndrome. The full effect of radiation is not apparent until the mature hematopoietic cells are depleted. Clinical symptoms during this period may include chills, fatigue, and petechial hemorrhage. Peripheral blood lymphopenia develops during the first 12 to 48 h after any significant exposure. Beyond 5 to 6 Gy, the rate and magnitude of the drop are not well correlated to radiation exposure. Some stem cells may survive acute exposure to >10 Gy. Death is from infection or bleeding and usually occurs before anemia can develop (red blood cell half-life is 100 to 120 days).

The $LD_{50/60}$ (the dose at which 50% of the population is dead by 60 days) is around 3.25 Gy if support is not given. There is considerable variability in the total-body dose tolerated. The very young and the old are more radiosensitive than middle-aged and young adult individuals. Females in general appear to be more tolerant of radiation than males. Persons exposed to <2 Gy will require little or no therapy but should probably be observed closely with daily blood counts for a few days.

The role of bone marrow transplantation for patients exposed to acute total-body irradiation is debated. At doses <8 Gy, the patient is likely to survive with supportive care. Most people exposed to doses higher than 10 Gy will die from the gastrointestinal syndrome. Therefore, 8 to 10 Gy may be the dose range in which bone marrow transplantation could have a role, although the Chernobyl experience did not confirm this prediction. Estimating the dose received by a given patient after radiation exposure is difficult. However, exposure estimation must be done quickly because bone marrow transplantation is most effective if it is performed within the first 3 to 5 days after exposure.

Acute Radiation Syndromes Following Whole Body Irradiation

Syndromes

Features	CNS	Gastrointestinal	Haemopoietic
Main organ affected	Brain	Small bowel	Bone marrow
Major pathology	Vasculitis, encephalitis, oedema (CNS)	Depletion of intestinal epithelium, infection	Bone marrow atrophy, pancytopenia, haemorrhage, infection
Threshold dose for onset (Gy)	20	5	1
Threshold dose for death (Gy)	50	10	2
Onset following exposure	0.25–3 hours	3–5 days	2–3 weeks
Typical clinical features	Lethargy, tremor, seizures, ataxia	Malaise, anorexia, nausea, vomiting, diarrhoea, fever, electrolyte imbalance,	Malaise, fatigue, exertional dyspnoea, leucopenia, thrombocytopenia, purpura
Time of death	Within 2 days	3–14 days	3–8 weeks

LATE RADIATION SIDE-EFFECTS

The late effects of radiation treatment develop gradually over several months or years. The changes that result may be sufficiently slight as to cause no clinical symptoms, or so rare as to present minimal risk to the individual. Nevertheless, the late changes that do occur warrant notice and care in all patients who have received radiation treatment. In those few individuals with serious late effects (generally less than 5% of patients who have received high-dose radiation) the results are often disastrous and treatment extremely difficult.

I. Scarring

Radiation treatment results in increased connective tissue, fibrosis and scarring often associated with atrophy of accessory tissues. This leads to some increased rigidity of tissues, less suppleness and less resistance to injury.

In addition, the walls of small blood vessels may be thickened and distorted, leading to reduction in blood supply to some tissues. This particularly leads to less ability to deal with injury or trauma such as that resulting from infection or surgery.

Any area of the body that has received radiation treatment should be treated "gently" for the rest of the patient's life.

II. Carcinogenicity

Radiation is one of the causes of cancer. Very rarely leukemia may result some five to twenty years after radiation exposure, due to bone marrow cells being damaged during radiation therapy. Similarly cancer can result in the area treated twenty or more years later. Historically osteo-sarcoma was seen in radium dial painters.

The chances of either of these occurring are very small indeed.

The patient's risk of dying of the original disease, unless successfully treated, are much higher than the risk of developing cancer from the treatment.

Nevertheless, the risk is there and is one of the reasons why benign diseases are not treated by radiation unless absolutely necessary.

III. Genetic Effects

Exposure of the gonads to radiation increases the risk of abnormal mutations and genetic changes. Most chromosome damage from radiation results in a failure of conception and not an abnormal child. Even if both parents have been exposed to radiation, the risks of abnormal children being produced are so small as to be almost negligible. Late genetic effects in the individual are much less important than the increased risk of inducing cancer or the late vascular changes produced by radiation treatment.

Typical dose to radiation workers
(Note: Many receive no measurable doses)

(Exposed surface)	50-1000 mrem/year (0.5-1 rem/year)
(Under lead apron)	1-20 mrem/year (0.001-0.02 rem/year)
(To embryo-fetus-under lead apron)	Less than 10 mrem during gestation

ALARA (As Low As is Reasonably Achievable). This means that the radiation exposures resulting from the practice must be reduced to the lowest level possible considering the cost of such a reduction in dose. Accepted radiation safety practice at the present time is ALARA – radiation doses to patients, radiation workers, and the general public should be as low as reasonably achievable.

ORGAN SPECIFIC RADIATION DAMAGE

Central Nervous System

Traditionally, the central nervous system (CNS) has been described as relatively resistant to radiation-induced changes. When the human brain is treated with standard fractionation (1.8 to 2.0 Gy/d), acute reactions are seldom observed.

Subacute CNS reactions to radiation treatment are more common. The clinical manifestations may include *Lhermitte's sign*, which is a self-limited paresthesia occurring with flexion of the neck. It is believed to be due to transient demyelination of the spinal cord following significant radiation exposure. It can be seen 1 to 3 months after completion of radiation treatment to the spinal cord. The frequency of Lhermitte's sign varies according to the type of radiation therapy and can be as high as 15% after mantle-field radiation. Mild encephalopathy and focal neurologic changes can occur after irradiation limited to the cranium. If radiation treatments to the brain are given at the same time that chemotherapeutic agents are administered, the effects can be more severe, presumably reflecting altered permeability to the drugs. The effect of cranial irradiation is believed to be secondary to radiation effects on the replicating oligodendrocytes and possibly on the microvasculature. Both clinical and radiologic changes may simulate tumor progression and can often pose diagnostic and treatment dilemmas.

Postirradiation pathology and associated clinical symptoms typically begin 6 to 36 months after radiation therapy and are related to the total dose and volume treated. Fraction size appears to be the most important variable affecting the rate of postirradiation brain necrosis. Neurocognitive changes can also be seen in children after cranial irradiation. The important pretreatment factors that predict the degree of late CNS effects include the age at which cranial irradiation was given and neurocognitive functional level at the time of treatment.

A unique late effect of cranial irradiation combined with chemotherapy, known as *leukoencephalopathy*, has been described in some patients. Leukoencephalopathy is a necrotizing reaction usually noted 4 to 12 months after combined treatment with methotrexate and cranial irradiation. Dementia and dysarthria may progress to seizures, ataxia, or death.

Transverse myelitis after radiation treatment is a spinal cord reaction similar to cerebral necrosis. This syndrome consists of progressive and irreversible leg weakness and loss of bladder function and sensation referrable to a single spinal cord level. Flaccid paralysis eventually occurs. Symptoms can occur as early as 6 months after radiation treatment, but the usual time to onset is 12 to 24 months. Lhermitte's sign does not correlate with transverse myelitis.

Skin

Skin reaction can be seen within 2 weeks of fractionated radiotherapy, a delay that correlates with the time required for cells to move from the basal to the keratinized layer of skin. The severity of the reaction depends on the skin dose per fraction and the total dose delivered to an area of skin. Erythema is observed, soon followed by dry desquamation. The skin at this time can be erythematous, warm, and sometimes edematous. The vessels in the upper dermis are dilated, and inflammatory infiltration with granulocytes, macrophages, eosinophils, plasma cells, and lymphocytes is noted.

When a severe skin reaction occurs, it is usually located where the beam strikes the skin tangentially. *Moist desquamation* consists of eruption of the epidermal layer. Healing is through reepithelialization from cells of less affected basal layers. When skin reactions are severe, treatment interruptions are needed to permit healing.

Dry desquamation is treated conservatively. Symptoms of dryness can be alleviated by advising the patient to wear only cotton fabric next to the affected skin and to refrain from the use of irritants of any kind. If treatment becomes necessary, hydrophilic agents that do not contain heavy metals are recommended. Petroleum jellies should not be used, as they may trap bacteria and increase the chance of infection. Moist desquamation is best managed by leaving the affected area dry and open to air.

A chronic reaction to radiation can be seen starting 6 to 12 months after irradiation. The epidermis is usually atrophic and may be more easily injured than normal skin. Interstitial fibrosis may also be increased. Hyperpigmentation of irradiated skin outlining the treatment field can be seen within a couple of months after completion of irradiation. This will fade gradually. The skin becomes thin, and hair loss may be permanent. Radiation therapy can induce second malignancies, which tend to be more aggressive than cancers arising in patients without significant radiation exposure.

Heart and Blood Vessels

When cardiac disease appears after radiation treatment, it is often difficult to tell to what extent the radiation treatment was causative. The pathogenesis of atherosclerotic heart disease is multifactorial. Exposure of a large heart volume to high-dose radiation therapy accelerates the development of coronary artery disease. Acute "pericarditis" may result from cardiac irradiation. The symptoms may include chest pain and fever, with or without pericardial effusion. This syndrome is usually self-limited and typically manifests itself a few months after treatment. **Asymptomatic pericardial effusion may be the most common manifestation of radiation-induced heart disease.** It is usually detected by chest X-ray and confirmed by an echocardiogram.

Most patients with symptomatic radiation-induced constrictive pericarditis will have received more than 40 Gy to a large portion of the heart. The risk increases significantly with cardiac doses greater than 50 Gy.

Chronic cardiac changes may have their onset from 6 months to several years after irradiation. The clinical symptoms may indicate chronic constrictive disease due to pericardial, myocardial, and endocardial fibrosis—a pancarditis. The clinical signs may include dyspnea, chest pain, venous distention, pleural effusion, and paradoxical pulse.

Lung

The clinical symptoms of radiation pneumonitis can be separated into early and late phases. During the early phase, clinical manifestations may include dyspnea, cough, and fever. Shortness of breath is relatively infrequent. It is more common to observe only the radiologic changes on a chest X-ray, without clinical symptoms. The clinical signs and symptoms of radiation pneumonitis may appear in 3 to 6 weeks if a large region of lung is irradiated to a dose above 25 Gy. An infiltrate outlining the treatment field may become evident on the chest X-ray. Radiation changes should not occur outside the treated field. Computed tomography can often help in distinguishing radiation pneumonitis from other causes of the infiltrate. The incidence of radiation pneumonitis can be reduced with careful treatment planning designed to lower the total dose given to the treated lung volume. Permanent scarring that results in respiratory compromise may develop if the dose and the volume of lung irradiated are excessive. Dyspnea and cough may be severe and debilitating.

Patients with symptoms of radiation pneumonitis may respond rapidly to glucocorticoids, but the medication has little effect on fibrotic changes. Glucocorticoids must be tapered very slowly to avoid rebound exacerbation of symptoms, which can prove lethal for some patients. Prophylactic administration of glucocorticoids is of no proven merit. Supportive care includes bronchodilators and oxygen at the lowest possible FIO_2.

Digestive Tract

Pathologic changes of the epithelial layer occur early during radiation treatments. The underlying submucosa may become edematous, with dilation of capillaries. Recovery from radiation damage can be expected within a few weeks after completion of radiation therapy, provided that sufficient numbers of stem cells are left. The radiorosponsiveness of the aerodigestive tract, like that of other structures, is not uniform but varies according to the location.

Patients often have symptoms from radiation exposure that are similar to other forms of acute gastritis. The clinical signs include epigastric pain, loss of appetite, nausea, and vomiting. Decreased gastric acidity is observed after 15 to 20 Gy of fractionated radiation therapy. The tolerance of the stomach to radiation is also aggravated by addition of systemic chemotherapy, such as 5-fluorouracil.

The germinal centers of the bowel mucosa are in the crypts of Lieberkuhn. Newly formed cells move upward along the walls of the crypts as transitional cells, undergoing maturation. The epithelial lining of the small bowel is the most rapidly renewed system in the human body and is completely renewed in 3 to 6 days. Within 12 to 24 h after the first dose of radiation therapy, pathologic evidence of dead cells are seen in the mucosal lining. Complete denudation of the mucosal surface rarely occurs during a regular course of radiation treatment because of the high capacity of the mucosa for regeneration. However, a focal area of erosion may be seen. The histologic appearance may be nearly normal within 2 to 3 weeks after radiation therapy.

Clinical manifestations of acute radiation enteropathy are nausea and vomiting, diarrhoea, and cramping pain. Relevant factors contributing to the pathogenesis of diarrhoea include malabsorption and alterations in the intestinal bacterial flora. The severity of symptoms, as in other anatomic areas, is proportional to the irradiated volume and the total dose.

Symptoms of chronic radiation enteropathy include diarrhoea, abdominal cramping, nausea, malabsorption, vomiting, and obstruction. Progressive fibrosis, perforation, fistula formation, and stenosis of the irradiated portion of the bowel can occur during the chronic phase of radiation enteropathy. Most clinical manifestations of chronic changes occur between 6 months and 5 years after radiation therapy.

Conservative noninvasive treatment can frequently control gastrointestinal symptoms. A low-residue or elemental diet may be beneficial. When nonsurgical treatment fails to relieve severe symptoms, surgical intervention is often indicated.

Bladder

Radiation injury to the bladder generally becomes symptomatic 3 to 6 weeks after the start of treatment, and symptoms usually subside 3 to 4 weeks after completion of radiation therapy. Patients often complain of increased frequency and dysuria. Cystoscopy often shows diffuse mucosal changes similar to those of acute cystitis. Sometimes desquamation and ulceration can be seen. Without infection, urinary symptoms are managed symptomatically. Concurrent chemotherapy with cytotoxic agents such as cyclophosphamide increases the severity of the acute bladder reaction.

The late effects of high radiation doses to the bladder may include interstitial fibrosis, telangiectasia, and ulceration. The blood vessels may be dilated and prone to rupture, resulting in painless hematuria. These changes are often difficult to distinguish from tumor recurrence and progression. A contracted bladder may result from doses in excess of 60 Gy.

Testes and Ovaries

In general, type B spermatogonia are exquisitely sensitive to the effects of radiation. The type A spermatogonia are thought to be more resistant because their longer cell cycle time allows considerable variation in radiosensitivity among different phases of the cell cycle. Sertoli cells and Leydig cells are less radiosensitive than the spermatogonia. Elevated levels of follicle-stimulating hormone (FSH) and luteinizing hormone (LH) have been observed after as little as 75 cGy. Doses as low as 10 cGy to the testicles may result in injury to the type B spermatogonia. The single dose required for permanent sterilization on normal human males is believed to be between 6 and 10 Gy. In normal human males, sperm count recovery requires 9 to 18 months after a fractionated dose of 8 to 100 cGy.

The radiation dose necessary to induce ovarian failure is age-dependent. A single dose of 3 to 4 Gy can induce amenorrhea in almost all women over 40 years of age. In young women, oogenesis is much less sensitive to radiation than is spermatogenesis in men.

Tolerance doses of normal tissues to conventionally fractionated irradiation

Tissue/organ	$TD_{5/5} - TD_{50/5}$ (Gy)
Testes	1–2
Ovary	6–10
Eye (lens)	6–12
Lung	20–30
Kidney	20–30
Liver	35–40
Skin	30–40
Thyroid	30–40
Heart	40–50
Lymphoid tissue	40–50

Contd.

Contd.

Bone marrow	40–50
Gastrointestinal	40–50
Vasculoconnective tissue	50–60
Peripheral nerve	65–77
Mucosa	65–77
Brain	60–70
Bone and cartilage	> 70
Muscle	> 70

PREGNANCY AND RADIATION

Possible Radiation Effects on the Conceptus
- Prenatal Death
- Growth Impairment
- Mental Retardation
- Congenital Malformations
- Childhood Cancer

Effect	Sensitive Period (Dates Post-Conception)	Possible Estimated Risk	Threshold Dose
Prenatal Death	1-14 days	5–10 rem	
Growth Impairment	8-15 weeks	20 rem	
Severe Mental Retardation	8-15 weeks	10–40 rem	1 in 250 per rem
Intellectual Deficit	8-15 weeks (effect questionable)	10 rem	loss of 1 IQ point for every 4 rem
Congenital Malformations	2-8 weeks	5-25 rem	
Childhood cancer	2nd & 3rd Trimester are less sensitive than 1st Trimester	1 in 2000 per rem	

Minimizing Radiation Exposure

I. Know where the radiation is and where it is coming from
- Very little radiation comes directly from the X-ray source—outside of the collimated primary beam – since the X-ray tube is surrounded by lead shielding. Therefore, most radiation you will receive will be X-rays scattered from the patient

(unless you place yourself within the direct primary beam from the X-ray tube). Scattered X-rays from the patient are most intense on the radiation entrance side of the patient.

- Very important. The amount of scatter produced is proportional to the collimated area. *Reduce the collimation to reduce the scatter!*

II. Keep your hands out of the primary beam
- If your hands might intrude into the primary beam, then wear lead gloves.
- The primary beam in fluoroscopy may be larger than what you see on the image monitor.

III. Distance
- Radiation intensity decreases as the distance squared. If the dose rate at 1 meter is 16 mrem/min, then the dose rate at 4 meters is only 1 mrem/min.
- If you must be in the patient room when the X-rays are activated, step away from the patient as much as possible.

IV. Time
- The dose increases as the amount of time you are exposed to the radiation increases.
- Minimize the amount of time that you are in the patient room when the X-rays are activated. Minimize the amount of time the patient is exposed to X-rays.

V. Shielding
- Your dose is reduced by placing an attenuating material between you and the source of X-rays.
- Shielding can involve placing another person between you and the source of scattered radiation.
- Personal Shielding Items:
  – Lead Apron
  – Thyroid Shield
  – Lead Gloves
  – Leaded Glasses.

The above normally have 0.5 mm lead equivalent, which allows approximately a 2% transmittance of incident radiation.

- Equipment and Room Shielding:
  – Lead shielding drapes on X-ray equipment or
  – Mounted on arm to ceiling
  – Portable radiation shields (on wheels)
  – Leaded glass windows
  – Leaded walls.

STEREOTACTIC RADIOSURGERY

Stereotactic radiosurgery is a method of delivering a high concentrated dose of radiation precisely directed at the abnormality for the purpose of stopping the growth, eliminating the abnormality or relieving symptoms caused by the abnormality. Stereotactic radiosurgery is not surgery in the conventional sense, as it does not require an operation whereby an incision is made.

The goal of stereotactic radiosurgery is to deliver enough radiation to destroy or stop the growth of a lesion previously defined by specialized imaging techniques without adversely affecting surrounding tissue.

Stereotactic radiosurgery may be performed using a linear accelerator or a Gamma Knife. Although there are many similarities, there are several differences.

Stereotactic Radiosurgery using a Linear Accelerator:

After a stereotactic frame is attached to the patient's head by pins, an MRI and CT are taken of the brain to determine the precise location of the tumor. If the patient has an AVM, an angiogram and CT are performed with the frame attached. Computer-guided dosimetry is specified to match the lesion. Lesions up to 3.5 centimeters in diameter may be treated. A cone that approximates the size of the lesion is placed in the collimator of the linear accelerator. Cones range in size from 12.5 mm to 40 mm.

The patient is placed in a supine (lying on back) position on the treatment couch of the linear accelerator. The head is secured to prevent movement while receiving treatment. Radiation is given to the lesion from different directions called arcs. A predetermined amount of radiation is delivered in an arc, and then the treatment couch is rotated as is the collimator housing the cone and a predetermined amount of radiation is given. This sequence continues until the therapy is complete. The number of arcs used varies from 4 to 6 or more and takes approximately 30 minutes.

Stereotactic Radiosurgery using a Gamma Knife

After a stereotactic frame is attached to the patient's head using pins, an MRI and CT are taken of the brain to determine the precise location of the tumor. If the patient has an AVM, an angiogram and CT are performed with the frame attached. The Gamma Knife consists of a sphere containing 201 Cobolt-60 sources. These sources are positioned so that the beams are targeted to a point within a cavity in the instrument where the patient's head is placed and covered by a helmet, which narrows the beams and shields the head from unwanted radiation. The radiation is controlled by the percentage of the 201 ports that are used, the number of exposures and the head position. Computer-guided dosimetry is specified to match the lesion. Different beam sizes are available by using different helmets with holes of various sizes. Lesions from 5 to 40 millimeters can be treated which takes about 30 minutes. By performing multiple exposures and by readjusting the helmet and head position, different lesion shapes can be achieved.

Used in

1. **Intracranial Tumor:** Stereotactic radiosurgery may be used for treatment of primary brain tumors such as meningiomas, pituitary adenomas, pineal tumors, acoustic neuromas, craniopharyngiomas and cancerous tumors that arise from brain cells such as anaplatic astrocytomas or glioblastomas.

   Tumors that travel to the brain from other parts of the body such as cancer from the lung, breast or skin may also be treated by this technique.

2. **Arteriovenous Malformation**

   Arteriovenous malformations (AVMs) may be treated by stereotactic radiosurgery. AVMs are present from birth. AVMs result from arteries being connected directly to veins. During development inside the mother's womb, the arteries do not divide into capillaries before joining veins. Without capillaries that reduce the pressure in blood vessels, the higher pressure inside the arteries may cause rupture or bleeding because the veins are not able to tolerate as high a pressure as arteries. Surrounding brain cells do not receive the proper amount of oxygen, which may result in scar tissue being formed as the surrounding brain tissue is deprived of oxygen. The patient may develop seizures.

3. **Trigeminal Neuralgia**

   Patients who suffer from trigeminal neuralgia (facial pain) and who have not experienced relief from medication and cannot or elect not to be treated with surgery or other techniques may receive stereotactic radiosurgery.

SECTION THREE

Section 4

Commonly Asked Questions

1. **Curie is unit for:**
   - A. Exposure
   - B. Absorbed dose
   - C. Degree of potential danger to health
   - D. Quantity of radionuclide disintegrating per second

2. **Subperiosteal erosion is seen in:**
   - A. Scurvy
   - B. Hyperparathyroidism
   - C. Hypoparathyroidism
   - D. Rickets

3. **'Onion peel' appearance on radiograph is seen in:**
   - A. Giant cell tumor
   - B. Ewing's sarcoma
   - C. Osteogenic sarcoma
   - D. Multiple myeloma

4. **Fraying at the ends of long bones is seen in:**
   - A. Rickets
   - B. Scurvy
   - C. Osteogenesis imperfecta
   - D. Congenital syphilis

5. **Flower vase appearance on IVP is seen in:**
   - A. Horseshoe kidney
   - B. Polycystic kidney
   - C. Pyonephrosis
   - D. Congenital megaureter

6. **Which one of the following contrast medium is used for IVP?**
   - A. Lipoidil
   - B. Dianosil
   - C. Sod. diatrizoate (Hypaque)
   - D. Conray—420

7. Osseous metastasis is most common if tumor is in:
   - A. Bronchus
   - B. Colon
   - C. Pancreas
   - D. Adrenal

8. First radiological sign of Crohn's disease in terminal ileum is:
   - A. Aphthoid ulceration
   - B. Pseudo sacculation
   - C. Cobblestone pattern
   - D. Thickening of bowel wall

9. In X-ray, jejunum has a pattern of:
   - A. Valvulae connivantes
   - B. Taenia coli
   - C. Reverse 3 sign
   - D. None of the above

10. In Scurvy, wimberger sign is best seen in:
    - A. Lower end of femur
    - B. Lower end of radius
    - C. Patella
    - D. Upper end of radius

11. Air bronchogram is seen in:
    - A. Lung abscess
    - B. Lung cavity
    - C. Pneumothorax
    - D. Consolidation

12. In tuberculosis in an AIDS patient the chest X-ray looks like:
    - A. Miliary shadow
    - B. Cavity
    - C. Consolidation
    - D. Collapse

13. 'Tram line' calcification seen in skull X-ray are characteristic of:
    - A. Congenital cytomegalovirus injection
    - B. Congenital toxoplasmosis
    - C. Craniopharyngioma
    - D. Sturge Weber Syndrome

14. Soap bubble appearance is seen in:
    - A. Osteoid osteoma
    - B. Osteochondroma
    - C. Osteoclastoma
    - D. Osteogenic sarcoma

SECTION FOUR

15. First radiological sign of ulcerative colitis is:
    A. Pseudopolyp formation
    B. Loss of haustrations
    C. Tubular colon
    D. Increased retrorectal space

16. Sunray appearance on X-ray is seen in:
    A. Osteogenic sarcoma
    B. Ewing's sarcoma
    C. Multiple myeloma
    D. Osteoclastoma

17. All of the following are radiological features of tuberculosis of spine except:
    A. Large paravertebral abscess
    B. Marked osteoblastic response
    C. Marked collapse of vertebra
    D. Deceased joint space

18. Multiple 'punched out holes' in skull are seen in:
    A. Hyperparathyroidism
    B. Multiple myeloma
    C. Thalassemia major
    D. Acromegaly

19. Best radiological view for diagnosis of fracture scaphoid is:
    A. Anteroposterior
    B. Lateral
    C. Oblique
    D. Any of the above

20. Osteosarcoma is differentiated from myositis ossificans by radiology by:
    A. Location
    B. Absence of osteomyelitic changes
    C. Shape of swelling
    D. Peripheral field of differentiation

21. Most common cause of 'target lesion' in stomach is:
    A. Melanoma   B. Carcinoid
    C. Lymphoma   D. Fibroma

22. Which of the following tumor is least sensitive to radiation:
    A. Bronchogenic carcinoma
    B. Adenocarcinoma of colon
    C. Malignant melanoma
    D. Osteogenic sarcoma

23. All are radiological features of ricket *except*:
   A. Ill defined epiphysis
   B. Narrow growth plate
   C. Frayed and widened metaphysis
   D. Metaphyseal cupping

24. Cobalt 60 is:
   A. Naturally occurring radioisotope
   B. Artificial radioisotope
   C. Product of plutonium
   D. Product of uranium

25. Safest light used in darkroom in a X-ray department is:
   A. Dull white
   B. Blue
   C. Green
   D. Red

26. Rat tail appearance is seen in:
   A. Achalasia cardia
   B. Reflux esophagitis
   C. Carcinoma oesophagus
   D. Hiatus hernia

27. In intravenous pyelography, one contracted kidney indicates:
   A. Hydronephrosis
   B. Polycystic kidney
   C. Chronic glomerulonephritis
   D. Chronic pyelonephritis

28. Best diagnosis of pancreatic cancer (head) is by:
   A. Ultrasound
   B. ERCP
   C. CT scan
   D. Angiography

29. Which of the following primary produces a Radio-opaque secondary in bone?
   A. Prostate   B. Thyroid
   C. Kidney   D. Breast

30. X-ray was discovered by Roentgen in:
   A. 1886   B. 1902
   C. 1895   D. 1907

31. In atresia of cardiac end of stomach, X-ray chest is best done with:
   A. Conray 240   B. Urograffin
   C. Barium sulphate D. Dianosil

SECTION FOUR

32. In phlebography dye is injected into:
    A. Anterior tibial vein
    B. Great saphenous vein
    C. Dorsal metatarsal vein
    D. Short saphenous vein

33. Absolute contraindication for IVP is:
    A. Idiosyncrasy to iodine
    B. Multiple myeloma
    C. Raised blood urea
    D. Bilateral ureteric obstruction
    E. All of the above

34. Best investigation for diagnosis of ampullary gall
    stone with obstructive jaundice is:
    A. Intravenous cholecystography
    B. OCG
    C. PTC
    D. ERCP

35. Investigation of choice for assessing a child with
    vesico-ureteric reflux is:
    A. Antegrade IVP
    B. Retrograde IVP
    C. Micturating cystourethrogram
    D. Cystoscopy

36. Best diagnosis of tracheo-oesophageal fistula is by:
    A. Barium sulphate
    B. Conray 240
    C. Dianosil
    D. Urograffin

37. Which of the following is not a radiological feature
    of meningioma?
    A. Lamellar calcification
    B. Enlarged foramen spinosum
    C. Increased meningeal vascular markings
    D. Decalcification inner table

38. Radium paint causes:
    A. Squamous cell carcinoma
    B. Osteogenic sarcoma
    C. Rodent ulcer
    D. Adenocarcinoma stomach

39. Best diagnosis of pancreatic cancer (head) is by:
    A. Ultrasound
    B. ERCP
    C. CT scan
    D. Angiography

40. **Honey comb appearance on X-ray is seen in all** *except*:
    A. Rheumatoid arthritis
    B. Tuberous sclerosis
    C. Histiocytosis X
    D. Wegener's granulomatosis

41. **X-rays are:**
    A. Electrons
    B. Protons
    C. Neutrons
    D. Electromagnetic waves

42. **Vessels catheterized on carotid angiography are:**
    A. 2 external carotids and 2 vertebral
    B. 2 internal carotids and 2 vertebral
    C. 2 internal carotids and 1 vertebral
    D. 2 external carotids and 1 vertebral

43. **Nucleus of an atom contains:**
    A. Electrons
    B. Only protons
    C. Electrons and protons
    D. Protons and neutrons

44. **Radium gives:**
    A. α-rays
    B. β rays and γ rays
    C. X-rays
    D. All of the above

45. **Isotopes have same atomic:**
    A. Number
    B. Weight
    C. Both weight and number
    D. Density

46. **Atomic weight is equal to total number of:**
    A. Protons
    B. Protons and neutrons
    C. Protons and electrons
    D. Protons, neutrons and electrons

47. **Egg shell calcification of hilar lymph nodes is most often due to:**
    A. Sarcoidosis
    B. Silicosis
    C. Abestosis
    D. Beryllosis

48. **In PA view of X-ray chest, right border of the heart is formed by all *except*:**
    A. Superior venacava
    B. Inferior venacava
    C. Right atrium
    D. Left atrial appendage

49. **All of the following dyes are water soluble *except*:**
    A. Metrizamide
    B. Iohexol
    C. Conray 420
    D. Myodil

50. **Nephrogram phase of IVP is because of dye in:**
    A. Proximal convoluted tubules
    B. Renal pelvis
    C. Nephron
    D. Collecting tubules

51. **Pneumothorax is best demonstrated by taking a radiograph, with patient in:**
    A. Mid inspiration
    B. End expiration
    C. Full inspiration
    D. Supine

52. **Double bubble sign is a radiological feature of:**
    A. Pyloric stenosis
    B. Duodenal atresia
    C. Hirschsprung's disease
    D. Necrotising enterocolitis

53. **The ½ life of CO_{60} is:**
    A. 2.6 years
    B. 5.2 years
    C. 8 years
    D. 3200 years

54. **Sign suggestive of carcinoma lung on chest X-ray is:**
    A. Rib erosion
    B. Central destruction within lesion
    C. Flattening of diaphragm
    D. Calcification

55. **Decreased teeth enamel is seen in all *except*:**
    A. Hyperparathyroidism
    B. Cushing syndrome
    C. Fluorosis
    D. Osteomalacia

56. **Unilateral hypertranslucent hemithorax on chest X-ray is seen in:**
    A. Bronchial asthma
    B. Fallot's tetralogy
    C. Pulmonary hypertension
    D. Poliomyelitis

57. **The dye used for OCG is:**
    A. Iopanoic acid
    B. Sodium diatrozite
    C. Biligraffin
    D. Meglumine iodothalamate

58. **For small pneumothorax, X-ray is done in:**
    A. Inspiration PA view
    B. Expiration PA view
    C. Lateral decubitus
    D. Supine

59. **Source of gamma rays is:**
    A. Radium
    B. Cobalt
    C. Cesium
    D. Xenon

60. **All are features of raised intracranial tension in adults *except*:**
    A. Erosion of dorsum sella
    B. Erosion of posterior clinoid process
    C. Inner table convolutions
    D. Sutural diastasis

61. **Cortical spur is found in:**
    A. Rickets
    B. Scurvy
    C. Hypervitaminosis
    D. Fluorosis

62. **Barium meal picture of carcinoma stomach shows:**
    A. Filling defect
    B. Loss of rugosity
    C. Small capacity of stomach
    D. Delayed emptying of barium
    E. All of the above

63. **X-ray changes in acromegaly are all *except*:**
    A. Lengthened terminal phalanx
    B. Widened joint spaces
    C. Obtuse angle of mandible and lengthening of mandible
    D. Premature osteoarthritis

SECTION FOUR

64. **Bronchography may be dangerous if a patient with:**
    - A. Emphysema
    - B. Bronchiectasis
    - C. Iodine sensitivity
    - D. All of the above

65. **Most common cause of punched out lesions in phalanges is:**
    - A. Enchondroma
    - B. Chondrosarcoma
    - C. Aneurysmal bone cyst
    - D. Multiple myeloma

66. **X-rays are formed when electrons hit:**
    - A. Water
    - B. Anode
    - C. Radium source
    - D. None of the above

67. **X-rays are produced by:**
    - A. Electrons
    - B. Neutrons
    - C. Positrons
    - D. Protons

68. **Which of the following is not an artificial radio isotope element?**
    - A. CO6O
    - B. I-125
    - C. Ra226
    - D. Tc99
    - E. Co59

69. **Pipe stem colon is seen in:**
    - A. Ulcerative colitis
    - B. Carcinoma colon
    - C. Crohn's disease
    - D. Whipple's disease

70. **Right sided pleural effusion is best viewed in which position:**
    - A. Left lateral decubitus
    - B. Right lateral decubitus
    - C. Full inspiration erect
    - D. Full expiration erect

71. **Spider leg deformity of calyces on IVP is seen in:**
    - A. Hypernephroma
    - B. Hydronephroses
    - C. Wilm's tumor
    - D. Pyelonephritis

72. **Calcification of the intervertebral disc is present in:**
    - A. Maple syrup urine disease
    - B. Homocystinuria

   C. Ankylosing spondylitis
   D. Achondroplasia

73. **Which of the following is not a radiological change in mucopolysaccharidosis?**
   A. J shaped sella turcica
   B. Spatulate ribs
   C. Anterior beaking of the vertebra
   D. Genu varum

74. **Ectopic pregnancy can be ruled out on ultrasound by:**
   A. Finding foetus in uterus
   B. Normal adenexa
   C. Uterus size proportional to foetal size
   D. Clinical examination

75. **Earliest radiological feature in rheumatoid arthritis is:**
   A. Decreased joint space
   B. Juxta articular osteoporosis
   C. Periarticular soft tissue swelling
   D. Subchondral erosions

76. **Pleural calcification is seen in:**
   A. Asbestosis
   B. Mesothelioma
   C. Pulmonary infarction
   D. Anthracosis

77. **Vesicoureteric reflux is best demonstrated by:**
   A. Intravenous pyelography
   B. Micturating cystourethrogram
   C. Retrograde pyelography
   D. Isotope renography

78. **Coiled spring appearance on barium enema is seen in:**
   A. Carcinoma colon
   B. Sigmoid volvulus
   C. Intussusception
   D. Ileal atresia

79. **Which of the following is not true about non contrast CT scan in head injury?**
   A. Subdural hematoma increase in density over lesional CT scans over weeks
   B. Extra dural haematomas are usually lens shaped
   C. Acute subdural hematoma appears as crescent shadow of increased density

SECTION FOUR

D. Subarachnoid haemorrhage appears as areas of increased density in basilar cisterns

80. **Widening of C-loop of duodenum/broad loop of duodenum on X-ray is diagnostic of:**
    A. Chronic pancreatitis
    B. Carcinoma head of pancreas
    C. Periampullary carcinoma
    D. Calculi in ampulla of vater

81. **Intraductal calcification of pancreas is seen in all *except*:**
    A. Tropical pancreatitis
    B. Alcoholic pancreatitis
    C. Hypoparathyroidism
    D. Kwashiorkor

82. **CSF on MRI appears:**
    A. Hyperintense on T_1 weighed image and hypointense on T_2 weighed image
    B. Hypointense on T_1 weighed image and hyperintense on T_2 weighed image
    C. Hyperintense on T_1 and T_2 weighed images
    D. Hypointense on T_1 and T_2 weighed images

83. **Chain of lakes appearance on ERCP is seen in:**
    A. Choledocholithiasis
    B. Chronic relapsing pancreatitis
    C. Traumatic pancreatitis
    D. Carcinoma head of pancreas

84. **Best view for right lung field will be:**
    A. Right anterior   B. Right posterior
    C. Left anterior   D. Left posterior

85. **Co-60 units:**
    A. γ radiation
    B. β radiation
    C. α and β radiation
    D. α, β, γ radiation

86. **Investigation of choice for diagnosis of Acute Pancreatitis:**
    A. USG
    B. Plain CT scan
    C. CT scan with contrast
    D. MRI Scan

87. **Investigation of choice for diagnosis of congenital hypertrophic pylori stenosis:**
    A. USG
    B. Barium meal

    C. Barium meal follow through

    D. CT scan with contrast

88. **Bird beak appearance of distal oesophagus is seen in:**

    A. Achalasia cardia

    B. Reflux oesophagitis

    C. Carcinoma oesophagus

    D. Hiatus hernia

89. **Contraindications to IVP is/are:**

    A. Idiosyncrasy to iodine

    B. Multiple myeloma

    C. Diabetes

    D. All of the above

90. **All of the following are features of splenic rupture on plain X-ray abdomen** *except*:

    A. Obliteration of psoas shadow

    B. Obliteration of splenic outline

    C. Obliteration of colonic air bubble

    D. Elevation of left hemidiaphragm

91. **Pulmonary thromboembolism on V-Q scan is suggested by:**

    A. Ventilation defect with normal perfusion

    B. Perfusion defect with normal ventilation

    C. Perfusion defect with ventilation defect

    D. Normal perfusion and ventilation

92. **Honey comb appearance on X-ray is seen in all** *except*:

    A. Wegener's granulomatosis

    B. Histiocytosis-X

    C. Tuberous sclerosis

    D. Rheumatoid arthritis

93. **Best parameter by USG to assess fetal maturity:**

    A. Crown rump length at 16 weeks

    B. Head circumference at 36 weeks

    C. Biparietel diameter at 12 weeks

    D. Femur length at 12 weeks

94. **Best imaging modality in patients with breast implants is:**

    A. MRI scan

    B. CT scan

    C. Mammography

    D. Radionuclide scan

SECTION FOUR

95. Minimal pleural effusion is best viewed in which position:
    A. Lateral decubitus
    B. Full inspiration erect
    C. Supine
    D. Full expiration erect

96. Earliest radiological change to appear in case of acute osteomyelitis is:
    A. Periosteal reaction
    B. Loss of plane between soft tissue and muscle
    C. Sequestrum formation
    D. Bony sclerosis

97. Calcification is best detected by:
    A. Plain X-ray
    B. USG
    C. CT scan
    D. MRI scan

98. 'Pseudokidney sign' on USG is seen in:
    A. Trichobezoar
    B. CA stomach
    C. CA kidney
    D. Polycystic kidney

99. Frequency of sound waves used for transabdominal ultrasonography is:
    A. 2.5-3.5 MHz
    B. 3.5-5.0 MHz
    C. 5.0-7.5 MHz
    D. 7.5-10 MHz

100. All of the following cause miliary shadow on X-ray chest except:
    A. Tuberculosis
    B. Histoplasmosis
    C. Coccidioidomycosis
    D. Wegener's granulomatosis

101. 'Telephone Handle' long bones are seen in:
    A. Achondroplasia
    B. Thanatophoric dwarfism
    C. Mucopolysaccharidosis
    D. Acromegaly

102. Which of the following is true about X-ray chest:
    A. Right hilum is lower than the left hilum
    B. Right dome of diaphragm is lower than the left

    C.   Pulmonary arteries normally extend upto the periphery of the lung field

    D.   All of the above

103. **Which of the following is Gold standard for the diagnosis of minimal bronchiectasis?**
    A.   Bronchography
    B.   Plain CT scan
    C.   X-ray chest
    D.   CT scan with contrast

104. **Which of the following cranial nerve can be visualised on plain CT scan?**
    A.   Optic
    B.   Trigeminal
    C.   Facial
    D.   Hypoglossal

105. **Radiosensitivity of tumour depends on:**
    A.   Histology
    B.   Blood supply
    C.   Nucleus atypia
    D.   Number of cells

106. **Speed of X-ray is equal to:**
    A.   Speed of light
    B.   Speed of electrons in X-ray tube
    C.   Tube voltage
    D.   All of the above

107. **Most radiosensitive phase of cell cycle is:**
    A. G_1 B. G_2
    C.   S   D.   M

108. **Popcorn calcification is seen in:**
    A.   Pulmonary hamartoma
    B.   Pulmonary hemorrhage
    C.   Pulmonary teratoma
    D.   Pulmonary embolism

109. **Nowadays radium is not used in the Rx of cancer because:**
    A.   It decays faster and needs frequent replacement
    B.   It decays into daughter Radon which is a constant hazard
    C.   It has a very long half life
    D.   It is a very unstable element

110. **The atom which scatters X-rays more is:**
    A.   Carbon
    B.   Mercury

C. Lead
D. Hydrogen

111. **Contrast in X-rays is dependent on:**
   A. KV
   B. mA
   C. Duration of exposure
   D. Distance between source and object

112. **In coarctation of aorta the rib changes are seen from:**
   A. 1-12th
   B. 3-6th
   C. 4-9th
   D. 8-12th

113. **Time sector imaging is preferred in infants because:**
   A. Child will be more co-operative
   B. Close to fontanelles
   C. Less expensive
   D. All of the above

114. **Time sector scanning of neonates is preferred because of the following reason most practical reason:**
   A. Open fontanelles
   B. Inexpensive
   C. Children more co-operative
   D. Better resolution

115. **Early change of pulmonary edema in CXR:**
   A. Batswing appearance
   B. Pleural effusion
   C. Kerley B lines
   D. Ground gram lung field

116. **Radiation is not used in:**
   A. CAT scan
   B. NMR
   C. Digital substraction imaging
   D. Thyroid scan

117. **The following is not an ionizing radiation:**
   A. MRI
   B. CT
   C. USG
   D. All are ionizing

118. **Hilar markings in a normal chest X-ray is formed by all *except*:**
   A. Pulmonary artery
   B. Bronchi

  C. Upper lobe veins
  D. Lower lobe veins

119. **Radiation mediates its effect by:**
  A. Denaturation of DNA
  B. Ionization of the molecules
  C. Protein coagulation
  D. Osmolysis of cells

120. **Pantomography is done for *except*:**
  A. Dental caries
  B. Dental cyst
  C. TM joint
  D. Transverse, fracture of Atlas

121. **Well defined lesion in the lung with pop corn calcification on X-ray is suggestive of:**
  A. Ca lung
  B. Adenoma
  C. Hamartoma
  D. Hydatid cyst

122. **Investigation of choice for a pregnant lady with upper abdominal mass:**
  A. Barium meal
  B. MRI
  C. CT scan
  D. DSA

123. **Well defined rounded opacity is the lung with cause irregular calcification is a feature of:**
  A. Hamartoma
  B. Hydatid cyst
  C. Amoebic abscess
  D. Ca lung

124. **The element used for intracavitary RT in carcinoma cervix:**
  A. Caesium
  B. Cobalt-60
  C. Strontium
  D. Radio iodine

125. **Investigation of choice for acute subarachnoid hemorrhage:**
  A. Enhanced MRI
  B. MRI
  C. CT scan
  D. Angiograpy

SECTION FOUR

126. 'Scalloping' of the edge of sigmoid colon on barium enema seen in:
    A. Diverticulosis
    B. Ulcerative colitis
    C. Carcinoma colon
    D. Pneumatosis intestinalis

127. Investigation of choice to differentiate pericardial effusion and dilatation of heart:
    A. Echocardiography
    B. Angio cardiography
    C. MRI
    D. CT

128. Least affected by radiation:
    A. GIT
    B. Gonads
    C. Cartilage
    D. Lymphocytes

129. Which of the following respond best to radiotherapy?
    A. Seminoma
    B. Teratoma
    C. Choriocarcinoma
    D. Endometrial carcinoma

130. Extent of cardiotoxicity of chemotherapy and radiotherapy is best diagnosed by:
    A. Echocardiogram
    B. Radionuclide scan
    C. ECG
    D. Endomyocardial biopsy

131. Ultrasonogram is not useful in:
    A. CBD stones at the distal end of the CBD
    B. Breast cyst
    C. Ascites
    D. Full bladder

132. Most serious complication of myelogram is:
    A. Allergy
    B. Transient neurological deficit
    C. Headache
    D. Arachnoiditis

133. Characteristics of benign tumor of lung in X-ray is:
    A. Size > 5 cm diameter
    B. Cavitation
    C. Peripheral location
    D. Concentric dense calcification

SECTION FOUR

134. **Extradural hematoma CT scan finding is:**
    A. Hypodense biconvex lesion
    B. Hyperdense biconvex lesion
    C. Concavo convex hyperdense lesion
    D. Low attenuated biconvex lesion

135. **Half life of Rn-222 is:**
    A. 3 days
    B. 3-6 days
    C. 4 days
    D. 5 days

136. **Mantle irradiation is used in:**
    A. Leukaemia
    B. Hodgkins disease
    C. Chest recondaries from some cancers
    D. Neuroblastoma

137. **In colour doppler the color depends upon:**
    A. Strength of returning echo
    B. Relation of transducer to blood flow
    C. Frequency of doppler used
    D. Type of doppler machine used

138. **Radioactivity was discovered by Becqueral in:**
    A. 1796   B. 1896
    C. 1901   D. 1946

139. **First investigation of choice for spinal cord tumor:**
    A. Myelography
    B. CT
    C. MRI
    D. Plain X-ray

140. **The patient who had dental extraction before radiotherapy needs:**
    A. No time for healing
    B. Adequate time for healing
    C. Radiotherapy is not advised
    D. Wait for one day to start radiotherapy

141. **Medusa lock appearance in X-ray is seen in:**
    A. Ascariasis
    B. Tapeworm
    C. Hook worm
    D. Ascaries and tapeworm

142. **One gray of radiation is equal to:**
    A. 1 rad
    B. 10 rad
    C. 100 rad
    D. 1000 rad

143. One of the following radioisotopes is used for interstitial thersapy:
    A. Phosphorus 32
    B. Iodine 131
    C. Iridium 191
    D. Gold 198

144. Diagnosis of aortic calcification is done by fluoroscopy by seeing:
    A. Side to side movement
    B. Up and down movement
    C. Combined movement
    D. None

145. For traumatic paraplegia investigation of choice is:
    A. MRI
    B. CT scan
    C. X-ray
    D. USG

146. CT findings of acute pancreatitis are all except:
    A. Dilatation of pancreatic duct
    B. Fuzzy outline of pancreas
    C. Parapancreatic fluid collection
    D. Edematous pancreas

147. Calcification in basal ganglia is seen in:
    A. Hypothyroidism
    B. Hypoparathyroidism
    C. Hypopituitarism
    D. Hypoaldosteronism

148. 'H' shaped vertebra is seen in:
    A. Phenylketonuria
    B. Sickle cell anemia
    C. Hemangioma
    D. Osteoporosis

149. Investigation of choice for multiple sclerosis:
    A. MRI
    B. CT scan
    C. X-ray
    D. EEG

150. Hydatid cyst of the lung in a chest X-ray:
    A. Is seen on calcified lung shadow
    B. Shows spackled calcification
    C. Will not calcify
    D. 1 and 2 are correct

151. **Cell most sensitive to radiation:**
    A. Lymphocyte
    B. Neurotrophil
    C. Basophil
    D. Platelets

152. **Deleterious effect of ultrasound on small organism is:**
    A. Ionisation
    B. Vacoulation
    C. Cavitation
    D. Disintegration

153. **CT scan was invented by:**
    A. Gedfrey Hounsfield
    B. Eric Storz
    C. John Snow
    D. Takashita Koba

154. **The first CT scan was manufactured by:**
    A. Hitachi, Japan
    B. Mitsubishi, Japan
    C. Electromusical instruments, England
    D. General Electric, USA

155. **The ½ life of I_{131} is:**
    A. 8 hours
    B. 2 days
    C. 5.2 days
    D. 8 days
    E. 12 days

156. **In diagnosis of acute myocardial infarction hot spot is seen with:**
    A. Thallium 201 scan
    B. Tc 99 scan
    C. Strontium 90 scan
    D. 1127 scan

157. **Parathyroid gland can be assessed by:**
    A. Thallium scan
    B. Technetium scan
    C. Gallium scan
    D. Plain X-ray neck
    E. Thallium technetium substraction scan

158. **Radio activity was discovered by:**
    A. Marie curie
    B. Pierre curie
    C. Rutherford
    D. Enrico formi
    E. Henri bequerel

SECTION FOUR

159. **String sign is seen in:**
    A.   Crohn's disease
    B.   TB of the ileocaecal region
    C.   Idiopathic hypertrophic pyloric stenosis
    D.   All of the above

160. **The substance used of OCG is:**
    A.   Iapanoic acid
    B.   Sodium diatrozite
    C.   Melglumine iodothalamate
    D.   Biligraffin
    E.   Dianosil

161. **Radiosensitising substances include:**
    A.   Oxygen
    B.   SR 250 8
    C.   Metronidazole
    D.   Misonidazole
    E.   All of the above

162. **Substance(s) which offer preferential radio-protection to tissues is/are:**
    A.   Cysteine
    B.   Thiophosphate WR 2721
    C.   Metronidazole
    D.   A and B are correct
    E.   Only C is correct

163. **Signs of increased intracranial tension in a child X-ray:**
    A.   Separation of the sutures
    B.   Tense anterior fontanelle
    C.   Silver beaten appearance of the bones
    D.   All of the above

164. **Commonly used type of radiation in radiotherapy is:**
    A.   Alpha rays
    B.   Beta rays
    C.   Gamma rays
    D.   X-rays

165. **Intracranial calcification in skull X-rays may be:**
    A.   Pineal calcifications
    B.   Dural calcifications
    C.   Cysticercosis
    D.   All of the above

166. **Notching of ribs on X-ray is seen in:**
    A.   PDA
    B.   ASD

C. Ebsteins anomaly

D. Coarctation of aorta

167. **Radiation protection shields are made up of:**

A. Copper

B. Silver

C. Lead

D. Tin

168. **Right border of the heart in a chest X-ray is not formed by:**

A. IVC

B. SVC

C. Right atrium

D. Aorta

169. **First sign after radiation R_x is:**

A. Erythema

B. Necrosis

C. Burns

D. Deep ulcer

170. **Isotope used in bone scans:**

A. Technetium

B. Gallium

C. Selenium

D. Chromium

171. **Abdominal organ best suited for CT scanning:**

A. Liver

B. Gall bladder

C. Pancreas

D. Kidneys

172. **Xeroradiography is used in... cancer detection:**

A. Stomach

B. Breast

C. Colonic

D. Pancreatic

173. **Pipe stem appearance in barium enema is seen in:**

A. Crohns disease

B. Ulcerative colitis

C. Schistosomiasis

D. Carcinoma colon

174. **Which tumour responds best to radiation?**

A. Poorly differentiated carcinoma

B. Anaplastic carcinoma

C. Well differentiated carcinoma

D. B and C

SECTION FOUR

175. **Micturating cystourethrogram is not used in:**
    A. Renal tumours
    B. Hydronephrosis
    C. Urinary obstruction
    D. Recurrent UTI

176. **Mammography is useful in:**
    A. Detection of early cancers
    B. Lobular carcinoma of opposite breast
    C. Large fatty breast
    D. All of the above

177. **Testicular tumour which responds best to radiation is:**
    A. Teratoma
    B. Seminoma
    C. Embryonal cell carcinoma
    D. None of the above

178. **Best investigation in acute cholecystitis is:**
    A. Technetium scan
    B. HIDA scan
    C. Pipida scan
    D. Plain X-ray abdomen

179. **The least radiosensitive tissue is:**
    A. Nervous tissue
    B. Bone
    C. Kidney
    D. Thyroid

180. **Cobalt60 is....radioactive source:**
    A. Artificial
    B. Natural
    C. Gamma ray
    D. Beta ray

181. **Left atrial hypertrophy is seen radiologically as:**
    A. Double cardiac silhoutte
    B. Left bronchial elevation
    C. Right ant. oblique view in barium swallow
    D. Left ant. oblique view in barium swallow

182. **Double bubble sign in an X-ray abdomen is indicative of:**
    A. Annular pancreas
    B. Ileal atresia
    C. Anal rectal malformation
    D. Duodenal atresia

183. Dye used in IV cholangiography is:
   A. Dianosil
   B. Conray
   C. Billigraffin
   D. Myodil

184. Percentage of cold thyroid nodules likely to be malignant:
   A. 20%
   B. 30%
   C. 40%
   D. 72%

185. Angle of tracheal bifurcation is increased in enlargement of:
   A. Right ventricle
   B. Left ventricle
   C. Right atrium
   D. Left atrium

186. Acute myocardial infarct scintigraphy is done with:
   A. Thallium
   B. Gallium
   C. Neodynium
   D. Tc stannous pyrophosphate

187. Hair on end appearance in skull X-ray is characteristic of:
   A. Sickle cell anemia
   B. Thalasemia
   C. Megaloblastic anemia
   D. Hemochromatosis

188. Intraosseous skeletal tumour is best diagnosed by :
   A. Plain X-ray
   B. NMR
   C. CT scan
   D. CT with scintiscan

189. The longest half life is that of:
   A. Radon
   B. Radium
   C. Uranium
   D. Cesium

190. Centenary year for X-ray is:
   A. 1995   B. 1999
   C. 1997   D. 2001

SECTION FOUR

191. **Most common cause of intracranial calcification is:**
    A. Pineal calcification
    B. Intracranial aneurysm
    C. Meningioma
    D. Tuberculoma

192. **Low dose radiotherapy is given for:**
    A. Seminoma
    B. Malignant melanoma
    C. Osteosarcoma
    D. Chondrosarcoma

193. **Obliteration of left heart border in PA chest X-ray is suggestive of:**
    A. Lingular pathology
    B. Left upper lobe lesion
    C. Left hilar lymph nodes
    D. Left lower lobe lesion

194. **The chest X-ray view best suites for pleural effusion detection is:**
    A. AP view
    B. PA view
    C. Lateral decubitus view
    D. Lateral view

195. **Investigation of choice to demonstrate vesico-ureteric reflex:**
    A. IVP
    B. Ultrasound
    C. Contrast MCU
    D. Cystoscopy

196. **The X-ray finding of small intestinal malabsorption syndrome are all except:**
    A. Increased transit time
    B. Mucosal atrophy
    C. Dilatation of bowel
    D. Flocculation of barium

197. **Kerley-B lines are seen when pulmonary venous pressure is:**
    A. 5 mmHg   B. 10 mmHg
    C. 20 mmHg   D. 40 mmHg

198. **Use of filters result in:**
    A. Softer beam radiation
    B. Wider beam coverage
    C. Less penetrating beam
    D. Beam of greater intensity

199. Use of a cone results in films of:
    A. Higher contrast
    B. Low contrast
    C. Less motion
    D. Long scale contrast
200. "Target material" which produces X-rays in a diagnostic X-rays tube is made of:
    A. Lead
    B. Tungsten
    C. Cobalt
    D. Copper
201. Point B in treatment of Ca Cervix by radiotherapy corresponds to:
    A. Obturator nodes
    B. Mackenrodts ligament
    C. Ischial tuberosity
    D. Round ligament
202. Dilatation of upper lobe veins is a reliable sign of:
    A. Cardiac decompensation
    B. Pulmonary ht.
    C. Emphysema
    D. Silicosis
203. Stryker's view is used in shoulder joint to visualise:
    A. Muscle calcification
    B. Recurrent subluxation
    C. Subacromial calcification
    D. Bicipital groove
204. "Marble bone" appearance is characteristic of:
    A. Osteopetrosis
    B. Osteogenesis imperfecta
    C. Fluorosis
    D. Achondroplasia
205. Latest source of neutrons for radiotherapy is:
    A. Strontium-90
    B. Iodine-131
    C. Calcifornium-256
    D. Radium-226
206. The radiological changes in Rickets are:
    A. Narrowing or absence of the normal zone of provisional calcification
    B. Fracture of the bone
    C. Epiphysis smaller than normal and have characteristic thin pencil line cortex
    D. Bowing of the bone

207. Causes of a cavitating lesion in the chest radiograph are all *except*:
    A. Hamartoma
    B. Pulmonary infarction
    C. Squamous carcinoma of the bronchus
    D. Caplan's syndrome
    E. Haematoma

208. The overall heart size in tetralogy of Fallot is usually:
    A. Markedly enlarged
    B. Normal or relatively small
    C. Slightly enlarged
    D. Moderately enlarged

209. The photo-sensitive material used in X-rays films consist of:
    A. Cellulose
    B. Silver bromide
    C. Zinc sulphide
    D. Cadmium tungstate

210. X-ray films are least sensitive to which coloured light:
    A. Violet
    B. Blue
    C. Yellow
    D. Red

211. The photo electric interaction occurs primarily in:
    A. 'L' cell
    B. 'K' cell
    C. Outer cell
    D. All shells equally

212. Normal metacarpal index is:
    A. Less than 5.4
    B. 5.4 to 7.9
    C. 8.4 to 10.4
    D. More than 10.4

213. Pericardial calcification is caused by all *except*:
    A. Radiotherapy to the mediastinum
    B. Methysergide therapy
    C. Anticoagulant therapy
    D. Benign pericarditis
    E. Dermatomyositis

214. **When bones show a 'Bone within bone' appearance this is indicative of:**
    A. Sickle cell anaemia
    B. Bone infarction
    C. Osteopetrosis
    D. Chronic myelogenous leukemia

215. **The "Target sign" ultrasonographically means:**
    A. Ovarian carcinoma
    B. Ectopic kidney
    C. Intussusception
    D. Liver metastasis

216. **In a modern rotatory anode X-ray tube cooling of anode is done by:**
    A. Conduction
    B. Convection
    C. Radiation
    D. All of the above

217. **"Champagne Glass" pelvis is seen in:**
    A. Achondroplasia
    B. Cretinism
    C. Down's syndrome
    D. Congenital dislocation of hip

218. **In ultrasound machines, the principle is:**
    A. Piezo electric crysial excitation
    B. Very low frequency radiowaves
    C. Microwaves
    D. None of the above

219. **Lymphangio myomatosis is characterized by all of the following *except*:**
    A. Post menopausal women
    B. Recurrent chylous pleural effusions
    C. Ascites
    D. Recurrent spontaneous pneumothorax

220. **"Golden S" sign is seen in:**
    A. Right upper lobe collapse
    B. Left upper lobe collapse
    C. Right middle lobe
    D. Lower lobe collapse

221. **"Grid" is a device which is used for:**
    A. Reducing scattered radiation
    B. Reducing patients exposure time
    C. Reducing the contrast of the X-ray
    D. All of the above

SECTION FOUR

222. **Estimation of foetal maturity by biparietal sonic measurement is accurate to within + -**
    A.   3-7 days
    B.   7-10 days
    C.   10-15 days
    D.   14-20 days
    E.   3-4 weeks

223. **Which of the following is diagnostic of the Rim sign' in a nephrogram?**
    A.   Pyelonephritis
    B.   Hyper nephroma
    C.   Polycystic kidney
    D.   Severe hydronephrosis

224. **Among the causes of rib notching are:**
    A.   Coarctation of aorta
    B.   Congenital interruption of aorta
    C.   Chronic superior venacava obstruction
    D.   Aortic arch syndrome
    E.   All of the above

225. **The following tumours of skin are radiosensitive, *except*:**
    A.   Cutaneous lymphoma
    B.   Basal cell carcinoma
    C.   Malignant melanoma
    D.   Squamous cell carcinoma

226. **In bone infarcts, all are true *except*:**
    A.   Dysbaric osteonecrosis are commonly juxta articular
    B.   Occur in Gaucher's disease
    C.   Occur in thalassaemia major
    D.   Are often diaphyseal in sickle cell disease
    E.   Are seen in acute pancreatitis

227. **The heart can be shifted to the left on the PA radiograph with:**
    A.   Sternal depression
    B.   Complete pericardial defect
    C.   Ventriculoseptal defect
    D.   Complete situs inversus
    E.   Marfan's syndrome

228. **Out of the following which is not a radiotherapy equipment?**
    A.   Betatron
    B.   Telecurie-cobalt unit

   C.   Linear accelerator
   D.   Thimble chamber
229. **Unit of one dose of radiation absorbed is:**
   A.   Grey
   B.   Roentgen
   C.   Curie
   D.   Bequerrel
230. **Thickness of stomach in ultrasound:**
   A.   2 mm
   B.   5 mm
   C.   7 mm
   D.   10 mm
231. **Thickness of lead apron to prevent radiation:**
   A.   1 mm
   B.   3 mm
   C.   0.5 mm
   D.   7 mm
232. **Presence of calcification in an intracranial lesion is best made out by:**
   A.   CT
   B.   MRI
   C.   Ultrasound
   D.   Contrast study
233. **Sunray appearance on X-ray is seen in:**
   A.   Ewing's sarcoma
   B.   Osteogenic sarcoma
   C.   Osteomyelitis
   D.   Condrosarcoma
234. **In aortic dissection the investigation of choice is:**
   A.   ECG
   B.   CT scan
   C.   Aortography
   D.   MRI scan
235. **Beheaded Scottish terrier sign is seen in:**
   A.   Spondylosis
   B.   Spondylolisthesis
   C.   Fracture transverse process of lumber vertebra
   D.   Fracture rib
   E.   Fracture scaphoid
236. **Isotope selectively concentrated in abscess cavities:**
   A.   Gallium
   B.   Technetium
   C.   Selenium
   D.   Chromium

237. **Egg shell calcification in hilar region is seen in:**
    A. Pneumoconiosis
    B. T.B.
    C. Sarcoidosis
    D. Aneurysms

238. **Left atrial enlargement is best seen with:**
    A. Chest X-ray AP view
    B. Chest X-ray left lateral view
    C. Barium swallow right anterior oblique view
    D. Barium swallow left anterior oblique view

239. **Radio-active gold is used in:**
    A. Bladder tumours
    B. Malignant ascites
    C. Gliomas
    D. None

240. **Radioactive phosphorous is used in treatment of:**
    A. Polycythemia
    B. Thyroid metastasis
    C. Multiple myeloma
    D. Embryonal cell carcinoma

241. **Unilateral elevation of diaphragm is commonly due to:**
    A. Obesity
    B. Large liver
    C. Scoliosis
    D. Congenital causes

242. **Isotope used for liver scan is:**
    A. Technetium
    B. I^{131}
    C. I^{132}
    D. Cobalt 60

243. **Radioactive cobalt emits:**
    A. Gamma rays
    B. Beta rays
    C. Alpha rays
    D. Neutrons

244. **Dead bone on an X-ray looks:**
    A. More radio-opaque
    B. Radiolucent
    C. Less radio opaque
    D. Is not seen at all

245. Pulmonary embolism is best diagnosed by:
    A. ECG
    B. Perfusion scan
    C. Angiography
    D. Plain X-ray

246. X-ray machine is kept at a distance of 6 feet from the photographic plate to:
    A. Magnify the image
    B. Prevent magnifications
    C. Enhance contrast
    D. None

247. Hot nodule is seen in:
    A. Adenolymphoma
    B. Mixed parotid
    C. Adenocystic carcinoma
    D. All

248. Most sensitive investigation of pancreatic carcinoma is:
    A. Angiography
    B. ERCP
    C. Ultrasound
    D. CT scan

249. Oligemic lung fields are seen in:
    A. TOF
    B. VSD
    C. ASD
    D. PS

250. Contrast material used in the diagnosis of esophageal atresia is:
    A. Barium swallow
    B. Gastrograffin
    C. Conray
    D. Dianosil

251. Which of the following are radioactive:
    A. CO 59
    B. CO 60
    C. I_{130}
    D. Yt 90

252. Target material used for generating X-rays:
    A. Tungsten
    B. Cobalt
    C. Cadmium
    D. Palladium

SECTION FOUR

253. **Widening of the C loop in X-ray is diagnostic of:**
    A. Chronic pancreatitis
    B. Carcinoma head of pancreas
    C. Periampullary carcinoma
    D. Calculi in the ampulla of water

254. **Hilar dance on fluoroscopy is seen in:**
    A. ASD
    B. TOF
    C. VSD
    D. TGV

255. **Water lilly appearance in chest X-ray is suggestive of:**
    A. Bronchiectasis
    B. Bronchopleural fistula
    C. Hydatid cyst
    D. Sequestration cyst of lung

256. **Dye used for myelography is:**
    A. Conray 320
    B. Myodil
    C. Dianosil
    D. Iopanoic acid

257. **Most sensitive test for metastatic deposit is:**
    A. Isotope scan
    B. CT scan
    C. Skeletal survey
    D. Tomography

258. **Echoencephalography is most useful for detecting:**
    A. Ventricular dilatation
    B. Midline shift
    C. Epilepsy
    D. Vascular lesions

259. **Echoencephalography is most useful in detecting:**
    A. Ventricular dilatation
    B. Midline shift
    C. Epilepsy
    D. Vascular lesions

260. **Isotope used in myocardial perfusion scan is:**
    A. Technetium
    B. Thallium
    C. Stannous pyrophosphate
    D. Gallium

SECTION FOUR

261. Echocardiography can detect pericardial effusion as little as:
    A. 15 ml
    B. 100 ml
    C. 150 ml
    D. 200 ml

262. Best diagnostic procedure in acute pancreatitis is:
    A. CT scan
    B. Ultrasound
    C. MRI
    D. Pipida scan

263. Most radio-dense substance is:
    A. Fluid
    B. Soft tissue
    C. Brain
    D. Bone

264. A neonate is brought with history of not having passed meconium on examination there is no anal opening but a dimple. Investigation of choice is:
    A. X-ray erect posture
    B. X-ray supine posture
    C. Gastrograffin study
    D. Invertogram

265. Isotope which is replacing radium is:
    A. Cesium
    B. Iridium
    C. Gold
    D. Californium

266. Acute radiation sickness is characterised by:
    A. Hematological symptoms
    B. CNS symptoms
    C. Gastrointestinal symptoms
    D. All of the above

267. Scottish terrier sign is seen in:
    A. AP view
    B. PA view
    C. Lateral view
    D. Oblique view

268. The tissue most resistant to radioactivity is:
    A. Rectum
    B. Colon
    C. Cervix
    D. Vagina

SECTION FOUR

269. **Least sensitive structure to radiation is:**
  A. Uterus
  B. Cervix
  C. GIT
  D. Vagina

270. **Newborn chest X-ray with respiratory distress shows multiple air containing lesions in left hemithorax and mediastinal shift is suggestive of:**
  A. Neonatal emphysema
  B. Diaphragmatic hania
  C. Pneumatoceles
  D. Congenital lung cysts

271. **Perihilar fluffy opacities on chest X-ray is seen in:**
  A. Pulmonary embolism
  B. Pericardial effusion
  C. Pulmonary arterial hypertension
  D. Pulmonary venous hypertension

272. **Best position for chest X-ray to detect left pleural effusion is:**
  A. Left lateral
  B. Supine
  C. Left lateral decubitus
  D. Right lateral decubitus

273. **Investigation of choice in traumatic paraplegia is:**
  A. MRI
  B. CT scan
  C. Ultrasound
  D. Beta rays

274. **Which is not mutagenic?**
  A. X-rays
  B. UV rays
  C. Ultrasound
  D. Beta rays

275. **Half life of Technetium 99 is:**
  A. 2 hours
  B. 6 hours
  C. 12 hours
  D. 24 hours

276. **Radiation exposure occurs in all *except*:**
  A. CT scan
  B. Plain X-ray
  C. Fluoroscopy
  D. MRI

277. The 'doughnut' sign seen on a brain scan usually suggests:
   A. Abscess
   B. Metastases
   C. Glioblastoma
   D. All of the above

278. Right lung is seen to best advantage on the following views:
   A. Right posterior oblique
   B. Right anterior oblique
   C. Left anterior oblique
   D. Lateral

279. Premature filling of veins is a manifestation in cerebral angiography of:
   A. Trauma
   B. Brain tumour
   C. Arteriovenous malformation
   D. Arterial occlusion

280. Widening of the C loop in X-ray is diagnostic of:
   A. Chronic pancreatitis
   B. Carcinoma head of pancreas
   C. Periampullary carcinoma
   D. Calculi in the ampulla junction

281. Lymphangitis carcinomatosa is a typical feature of:
   A. Carcinoma of the thyroid
   B. Carcinoma of the bronchus
   C. Hepatoma
   D. Hypernephroma
   E. Carcinoma of the pancreas

282. Renal scan should be done in which position:
   A. Supine
   B. Prone
   C. Sitting
   D. Left lateral

283. Ideal imaging modality to diagnose hydrocephalus in a one month old baby is:
   A. Plain X-ray
   B. Ultrasound
   C. Computerised tomography
   D. Magnetic Resonance Imaging

284. Biconvex hyperdense shadow on non-contrast CT scan is seen in:
   A. Extradural haemorrhage
   B. Subdural haemorrhage

C. Subarachnoid haemorrhage

D. Intraventricular haemorrhage

285. **A young female presents with chest pain not associated with exercise. Auscultation reveals multiple ejection clicks with a murmur. The most important investigation for diagnosis is:**
   A. ECG
   B. Thallium 201 scan
   C. Tc pyrophosphate scan
   D. Echocardiography

286. **A patient presents with ARF with a normal ultra-sound report. The next most useful investigation is:**
   A. Renal angiography
   B. Retrograde pyelography
   C. Intravenous pyelography
   D. DTPA scan

287. **Intracavitary radiation is given in :**
   A. Carcinoma of the cervix
   B. Carcinoma of the lung
   C. Carcinoma of the oesophagus
   D. Carcinoma of the oral cavity

288. **In a patient with renal cell carcinoma with a thrombus in the IVC-renal vein, which of the following is the best for diagnosis:**
   A. CT scan
   B. Angiography
   C. Colour Doppler imaging
   D. IVP

289. **Ultrasound detects all the following *except*:**
   A. Anencephaly
   B. Down syndrome
   C. Placenta praevia
   D. Hydatidiform mole

290. **An elderly man presents with a history of jaundice and pain abdomen. The investigation of choice is:**
   A. Ultrasound
   B. 4-quadrant aspiration
   C. CT scan
   D. X-ray abdomen

291. **The following chest X-ray findings are all suggestive of malignancy *except*:**
   A. Umbilicated surface
   B. Spiculated surface

    C. Peripheral cavitation

    D. Diffuse calcification

292. Antenatal diagnosis of hydrocephalus is done by:

    A. USG

    B. AFP estimation

    C. Foetoscopy

    D. Aminocentesis

293. Rib notching is seen in all the following *except*:

    A. Blalock-Taussing shunt

    B. Coarctation of the aorta

    C. IVC obstruction

    D. Neurofibromatosis

    E. None

294. A chronic smoker presents with complaints of haemoptysis. Chest X-ray appears to be normal. What is the next best investigation:

    A. Bronchoscopy

    B. High resolution CT

    C. Sputum cytology

    D. Bronchoalveolar lavage

295. All the following are radiological features of mitral stenosis except:

    A. Straight left heart border

    B. Oligaemia of the upper lung fields

    C. Pulmonary haemosiderosis

    D. Lifting of the left bronchus

296. Features of a benign lung lesion are:

    A. Speckled calcification

    B. Peripheral calcification

    C. Ring enhancement

    D. Shows hot spot with radio labelling agent

297. A 50-year-old male patient having a history of chronic smoking presents with a single lymph node enlargement and hoarseness of voice. The next line of management is:

    A. FNAC

    B. IDL with CXR

    C. Percutaneous biopsy

    D. Advise him very seriously to stop smoking

298. 'Tram-track calcification' in the brain is seen in:

    A. Sturge-Weber syndrome

    B. Toxoplasmosis

    C. Tuberous sclerosis

    D. Syphilis

SECTION FOUR

299. B/L symmetrical Hilar lymphnode seen in:
  A. Sarcoidosis
  B. Tuberculosis
  C. Leprosy
  D. Wegener's granulomatosis

300. The most sensitive and specific investigation in renal artery hypertension is:
  A. Captopril-enhanced renal scan
  B. Doppler ultrasound
  C. MRI
  D. CT scan

301. A patient has calcification on AP view of Right side of abdomen. In lateral view, calcification is seen to overlie the spine. The most likely diagnosis is:
  A. Gall stone
  B. Calcified mesenteric nodes
  C. Renal stones
  D. Calcification in vertebral sphenoid process

302. Most radiosensitive of the following is:
  A. Ca cervix   B. Ca kidney
  C. Ca Ovary   D. Ca Pancreas

303. Medullary cystic disease of the kidney is best diagnosed by:
  A. USG
  B. Renogram
  C. Nuclear scan
  D. Urography

304. Maximum penetration is seen with:
  A. α particles
  B. β particles
  C. γ particles
  D. Electron beam

305. The Radiological feature of Pindborg's tumour is:
  A. Onion-peel appearance
  B. Sun burst appearance
  C. Driven snow appearance
  D. Cherry blossom appearance

306. Characteristic finding in CT scan of patient with tubercular meningitis is:
  A. Exudates seen in basal cistern
  B. Hydrocephalus is not seen
  C. Ventriculitis
  D. Calcification in cerebellum

307. A neonate has a mass in kidney. USG shows hypoechoic shadow. The most likely diagnosis is:
   A. Wilm's tumour
   B. Neuroblastoma
   C. Mesonephroblastic tumour
   D. Adenoma

308. A 60-year-old man with suspected Bronchogenic carcinoma. TB has been ruled out in this patient. Investigation to be done in this patient is:
   A. CT guided FNAC
   B. Bronchoscopy and biopsy
   C. Sputum cytology
   D. Chest X-ray

309. Multiple punched out lesions on X-ray is seen in:
   A. Paget's disease
   B. Craniopharyngioma
   C. Multiple myeloma
   D. Eosinophilic granuloma

310. An obese patient has heavy, thick bones. A good X-ray is taken with:
   A. Increase in mA
   B. Increase in KVP
   C. Increased exposure time
   D. Increased developing time

311. All of the following are true about loculated pleural effusion except:
   A. It makes an obtuse angle with the chest wall
   B. The margins are clear when viewed in face
   C. Not confined to any broncho pulmonary segment
   D. Air bronchogram is seen within the opacity

312. All of the following are correct about radiological evaluation of a patient with cushing's syndrome except:
   A. MRI of the sella tursica will identify the cause of cushing's syndrome
   B. MRI of the adrenal glands may distinguish adrenal adenoma from carcinoma
   C. Adrenal CT scan distinguishes adrenal tumour from cortical hyperplasia
   D. Petrosal sinus sampling is the best way to distinguish the tumour from an ectopic ACTH producing tumour

313. **The investigation of choice in Aortic dissection is:**
    A. USG
    B. CT
    C. MRI
    D. Digital segmental angiography

314. **Pulmonary embolism is diagnosed by:**
    A. USG
    B. X-ray chest
    C. Ventilation perfusion scan
    D. CT scan

315. **"Chain of lakes" appearance on X-ray is seen in :**
    A. Chronic pancreatitis
    B. Acute pancreatitis
    C. Carcinoma head of pancreas
    D. Adenocarcinoma

316. **Investigation of choice for Acute subarachnoid haemorrhage is:**
    A. MRI
    B. Enhanced MRI
    C. CT scan
    D. Angiography

317. **On X-ray, right border of the mediastinum is formed by all the following *except*:**
    A. Superior vena cava
    B. Right atrium
    C. Right ventricle
    D. Right brachiocephalic vein

318. **Popcorn calcification is seen in:**
    A. Pulmonary hamartoma
    B. Fungal infection
    C. Metastasis
    D. Tuberculosis

319. **Best investigation for pericardial effusion is:**
    A. Cardiac catheterization
    B. USG
    C. Echocardiography
    D. Lateral view X-ray chest

320. **Investigation of choice in obstructive jaundice is:**
    A. ERCP
    B. Ultrasound
    C. Cholecystography
    D. X-ray

SECTION FOUR

321. **In MRI, strength of magnetic field is:**
   A. 0.5 Tesla
   B. 1.1 Tesla
   C. 5 Tesla
   D. 11 Tesla

322. **The principle used in Radiotherapy is:**
   A. Cytoplasmic coagulation
   B. Ionising the molecules
   C. DNA damage
   D. Low dose causes tissue necrosis

323. **The most common presentation of Radiation carditis is:**
   A. Pericardial effusion
   B. Atheromatous plaques
   C. Myocardial fibrosis
   D. Pyogenic pericarditis

324. **Which of the following is not done in a case of Brain tumour?**
   A. CT scan
   B. MRI
   C. X-ray skull
   D. Lumbar puncture

325. **Most common skin manifestation of radiotherapy:**
   A. Erythema
   B. Atopy
   C. Hyperpigmentation
   D. Dermatitis

326. **The most sensitive cell cycle stage for radiotherapy is:**
   A. S phase
   B. G_1
   C. G_2
   D. G_2M

327. **Ionising radiation acts on tissue depending upon:**
   A. Linear acceleration energy
   B. Excitation of electron from orbit
   C. Formation of pyrimidine dimers
   D. Thermal injury

328. **The most sensitive investigation for air embolism is:**
   A. Deceased tidal volume of CO_2
   B. Doppler
   C. Decreased tidal volume of NO_2
   D. Central venous pressure

329. Cardiotoxicity caused by radiotherapy and chemotherapy is best detected by:
    A. Echocardiography
    B. Endomyocardial biopsy
    C. ECG
    D. Radionuclide scan

330. Impaired renal function is assessed by:
    A. DTPA
    B. DMSA scan
    C. Iodohippurate
    D. MAGS

331. In cerebral angiography, dye is injected through:
    A. Femoral artery
    B. Brachial artery
    C. Axillary artery
    D. Radial artery

332. All of the following are used in Interstitial brachytherapy *except*:
    A. CO^{60}
    B. Ir^{192}
    C. Au^{198}
    D. CS^{137}

333. 'Figure of 8' appearance is seen in:
    A. TAPVC
    B. Partial TAPVC
    C. Abnormal origin of aorta
    D. Tetralogy of fallot

334. X-ray findings in cardiac failure are all of the following *except*:
    A. Kerley B lines
    B. Pleural effusion
    C. Prominent lower lobe veins
    D. Cardiomegaly

335. A 55-year-old male has a 5 cm cavitating lesion of unknown duration at the apex of the right lung. The investigation to be carried out:
    A. CT scan
    B. FNAC
    C. Bronchography
    D. Trans bronchial biopsy

336. Prominent left border of heart is formed by all the following *except*:
    A. Azygous vein
    B. Pericardial cyst

  C. Coronary artery aneurysm
  D. Enlarged left auricular aneurysm

337. **Radiological investigation in females of reproductive age should be restricted to :**
  A. First 10 days of menstrual cycle
  B. Last 10 days of menstrual cycle
  C. 10-20th day of menstrual cycle
  D. Period of menstruation

338. **Radiation exposure occurs in all of the following *except*:**
  A. CT scan
  B. MRI
  C. Fluoroscopy
  D. Plain X-ray

339. **Investigation of choice in parathyroid pathology is:**
  A. CT scan
  B. Gallium scan
  C. Thallium scan
  D. Technetium-thallium subtraction scan

340. **The earliest evidence of Rickets is seen by:**
  A. Radiological examination of growing end of bone
  B. S. alkaline phosphatase level
  C. S. calcium level
  D. S. phosphorus level

341. **The right side of mediastinum shadow is not formed by:**
  A. Superior vena cava
  B. Right innominate vein
  C. Right atrium
  D. Right ventricle

342. **The best view for visualising the sella turcica in X-ray is:**
  A. AP views
  B. Oblique view
  C. Open mouth view
  D. Lateral view

343. **Investigation of choice for small intestine tumor:**
  A. Ba meal follow through
  B. Echo
  C. X-ray abdomen
  D. CT scan with contrast

SECTION FOUR

344. **Acoustic shadow on USG is due to:**
   A. Reflection
   B. Refraction
   C. Artefact
   D. Absorption of waves

345. **The earliest congenital malformation that can be detected on USG:**
   A. Anencephaly
   B. Hydrocephalus
   C. Sacral agenesis
   D. Down's syndrome

346. **The best investigation for cardiac tamponade is:**
   A. 2-D echocardiography
   B. Real time echocardiography
   C. Ultrasound
   D. M-mode echocardiography

347. **The earliest sign of foetal life is best detected by :**
   A. Doppler
   B. Rcal time ultrasound
   C. Fetoscopy
   D. X-ray

348. **Increased radioisotopes are seen in all of the following *except*:**
   A. Primary bone tumour
   B. Osteomyelitis
   C. Paget's disease
   D. Pseudo arthrosis

349. **All of the following are radiological features of scleroderma *except*:**
   A. Diffuse periosteal reaction
   B. Oesophageal dysmotility
   C. Erosion of the tip of the phalanges
   D. Lung nodules

350. **Calcification of meniscal cartilage is feature of:**
   A. Acromegaly
   B. Hyperparathyroidism
   C. Reiter's syndrome
   D. Pseudogout

351. **Bilateral spider leg sign on IVP is suggestive of:**
   A. Polycystic kidney
   B. Hydronephrosis
   C. Hypernephroma
   D. Renal stones

352. All the following are features of radiation *except*:
    A. Fluorescein
    B. Biological
    C. Photographic
    D. Non penetrating

353. All the following show miliary shadows on chest X-ray *except*:
    A. Pneumoconiosis
    B. Mitral stenosis
    C. Sarcoidosis
    D. Staphylococcal pneumonia

354. Increased radiolucency of one sided hemithorax may be caused by all the following *except*:
    A. Obstructive emphysema
    B. Pneumothorax
    C. Expiratory film
    D. Rotation

355. An ideal imaging method for diagnosing hydrocephalus in an infant is:
    A. Plain X-ray
    B. CT scan
    C. Ultrasound
    D. MRI

356. IVP should be cautiously performed in:
    A. Multiple myeloma
    B. Bone secondaries
    C. Neuroblastoma
    D. Leukemia

357. Best method for detecting minimal bronchiectasis is:
    A. Bronchogram
    B. CT scan
    C. Radionuclide lung scan
    D. Chest X-ray

358. Investigation of choice to demonstrate vesico-ureteral reflux is:
    A. Isotope cystogram
    B. Contrast MCU
    C. IVP
    D. Cystoscopy

359. In perinatal asphyxia, neurological damage can be predicted by:
    A. Routine radiology
    B. CT

C. MRI

D. USG

360. **In intervertebral disc prolapse, schmorl node on MRI implies:**
    A. Significant
    B. Not significant
    C. Good prognosis
    D. Not prognostic

361. **CT scan shows a subarachnoid haemorrhage following symptoms of sudden headache and paralysis. Next investigation of choice is:**
    A. 4-vessel angiography
    B. SPECT
    C. Transacromial Doppler USG
    D. MRI

362. **The best method to diagnose bronchiectasis:**
    A. X-ray
    B. Bronchography
    C. MRI
    D. HRCT

363. **The posterior iliac horn is characteristic of:**
    A. Nail-patella syndrome
    B. Marfan's syndrome
    C. Hurler syndrome
    D. Acromegaly

364. **All are seen in left atrium enlargement *except*:**
    A. Posterior displacement of the oesophagus on barium meal
    B. Straightening of the left main bronchus
    C. A double shadow of right atrium
    D. Retrosternal lucency on lateral film

365. **The best investigation for parameningeal rhabdomyosarcoma:**
    A. CSF cytology
    B. MRI
    C. CECT
    D. SPECT scan

366. **Coarse 'Popcorn' calcification on mammogram is due to:**
    A. Fibroadenoma
    B. Fat necrosis
    C. Carcinoma in situ
    D. Phylloides tumour

367. **In a patient with renal cell carcinoma with a thrombus in IVC renal vein, which is the best investigation for diagnosis:**
    - A. CT scan
    - B. Angiography
    - C. Colour doppler imaging
    - D. IVP

368. **Radiofrequency ablation treatment is most useful in:**
    - A. Ventricular fibrillation
    - B. Atrial fibrillation
    - C. WPW syndrome
    - D. Ventricular premature complex

369. **The X-ray appearance of a CBD stone on cholangiography is:**
    - A. Meniscus appearance
    - B. Eccentric occlusion
    - C. Sudden cut off
    - D. Smooth tapering

370. **Epiphyseal enlargement is seen in:**
    - A. Rickets
    - B. Ankylosing spondylitis
    - C. Spondo-epiphyseal dysplasia
    - D. Juvenile rheumatoid arthritis

371. **On X-ray of the abdomen, soap bubble appearance is seen in:**
    - A. Multiple cystic kidney
    - B. Meconium ileus
    - C. Cystic lymphangiectasis
    - D. Volvulus

372. **Medusa head appearance on abdominal X-ray indicates:**
    - A. Roundworm
    - B. Tapeworm
    - C. Roundworm and tape worm
    - D. Amoebiasis

373. **Which of the following is a less useful diagnostic procedure in a case of Acute haematemesis?**
    - A. Barium meal
    - B. Endoscopy
    - C. Gastric content aspiration
    - D. Angiography

SECTION FOUR

374. The method to diagnose displaced intra-uterine device is:
   A. Ultrasound
   B. X-ray abdomen (erect view)
   C. Uterine sound and hysteroscopy
   D. All of the above

375. The most common calcifying brain tumour in a child is:
   A. Medulloblastoma
   B. Craniopharyngioma
   C. Glioma
   D. Meningioma

376. Geographic lytic lesions in the vault of the skull with bevelled edges are seen with:
   A. Eosinophilic granuloma
   B. Multiple myeloma
   C. Hyperparathyroidism
   D. Reticular cell carcinoma

377. Which of the following is most radiosensitive tumour?
   A. Astrocytoma
   B. Medulloblastoma
   C. Craniopharyngioma
   D. Teratoma

378. 'Cavitating lesions' in the lung are found in:
   A. Squamous cell carcinoma
   B. Adenocarcinoma
   C. Small cell carcinoma
   D. Large cell carcinoma

379. Which of the following is most radioresistant?
   A. Cartilage
   B. GIT epithelium
   C. Gonadal tumours
   D. Ewing's sarcoma

380. Which of the following is the most radiosensitive ovarian tumour?
   A. Endodermal sinus tumour
   B. Dermoid cyst
   C. Dysgerminoma
   D. Serous cyst adenoma

381. The most important investigation for posterior urethral value is:
   A. Urethroscopy
   B. IVP

    C. Retrograde cystogram

    D. Micturating cystogram

382. **The X-ray view for supra orbital fissure is:**

    A. Towne's   **B.** Caldwell

    C. AP   **D.** Basal

383. **In scurvy all of the following radiological signs are seen *except*:**

    A. Pelican spur

    B. Soap bubble appearance

    C. Zone of demarcation near epiphysis

    D. Frenkel's line

384. **On radiography widened duodenal 'C' loop with irregular mucosal pattern on upper gastrointestinal barium series is most likely due to:**

    A. Chronic pancreatitis

    B. Carcinoma head of pancreas

    C. Duodenal ulcer

    D. Duodenal ileus

385. **A young man with pulmonary tuberculosis presents with massive recurrent hemoptysis. For angiographic treatment, which vascular structure should be evaluated first:**

    A. Pulmonary artery

    B. Bronchial artery

    C. Pulmonary vein

    D. Superior venacava

386. **In which of the following a 'Cour-en-Sabot' shape of the heart is seen:**

    A. Tricuspid atresia

    B. Ventricular septal defect

    C. Transposition of great arteries

    D. Tetralogy of Fallot

387. **A 55-year-old man, who has been on bed rest for the past 10 days, complains of breathlessness and chest pain. The chest x-ray is normal. The next step in investigation should be:**

    A. Lung Ventilation - perfusion scan

    B. Pulmonary arteriography

    C. Pulmonary venous wedge angiography

    D. Echocardiography

388. **Which of the following brain tumors does not spread via CSF?**

    A. Germ cell tumors

    B. Medulloblastoma

SECTION FOUR

C.   CNS Lymphoma

D.   Craniopharyngioma

389. **Which of the following is not an indication of RT in Pleomorphic adenoma of parotid?**

A.   Involvement of deep lobe

B.   2nd histologically benign recurrence

C.   Microscopically positive margins

D.   Malignant transformation

390. **Which of the following is the most penetration beam?**

A.   Electron beam   B.   8 MV photons

C.   18 MV photons   D.   Proton beam

391. **The radiation tolerance of whole liver is:**

A.   l5 Gy   B.   30 Gy

C.   40 Gy   D.   45 Gy

392. **A 25 yr old man presented with fever, cough, expectoration, and breathlessness of 2 months duration. Contrast enhanced computed tomography of chest showed bilateral upper lobe fibrotic lesions and mediastinum has enlarged necrotic nodes with peripheral rim enhancement. Which one of the following is the most probable diagnosis?**

A.   Sarcoidosis

B.   Tuberculosis

C.   Lymphoma

D.   Silicosis

393. **Which of the following radioisotopes is commonly used as a source for external beam radiotherapy in the treatment of cancer patients:**

A.   Strontium-89

B.   Radium-226

C.   Cobalt-59

D.   Cobalt-60

394. **Which of the following is the best choice to evaluate radiologically a posterior fossa tumor?**

A.   CT scan

B.   MRI

C.   Angiography

D.   Myelography

395. **A patient is suspected to have vestibular Shwanomma, The investigation of choice for its diagnosis is:**

A.   Contrast enhanced CT scan

B.   Gadolinium enhanced MRI

C. SPECT

D. PET scan

396. **Radiological findings in meningioma are all** *except*:
    A. Calcification
    B. Vascular markings
    C. Osteosclerosis
    D. None of the above

397. **Superior orbital fissure best view is:**
    A. Plain AP view
    B. Caldwell
    C. Townes
    D. Basal view

398. **Best diagnosis for dissecting aorta is:**
    A. CT scan
    B. MRI
    C. Angiography
    D. X-ray

399. **The causes of homogenous opacity on X-ray is all** *except*:
    A. Pleural effusion
    B. Diaphragmatic hernia
    C. Massive consolidation
    D. Emphysema

400. **About osteogenesis imperfecta; all are true** *except*:
    A. Diaphyseal fractures
    B. Metaphyseal fractures
    C. Classified by sillence classification
    D. Scleral and dental abnormalities

401. **For the evaluation of blunt abdominal trauma which of the following imaging modalities is ideal?**
    A. Ultrasonography
    B. Computed tomography
    C. Nuclear scintigraphy
    D. Magnetic resonance imaging

402. **Following are common features of malignant gastric ulcer on barium meal** *except*:
    A. Location on the greater curvature
    B. Carman's meniscus sign
    C. Radiating folds which do not reach the edge of the ulcer
    D. Lesser curvature ulcer with a nodular rim

403. **What dose of radiation therapy is recommended for pain relief in bone metastases?**
   A. 8 Gy in one fraction
   B. 20 Gy in 5 fractions
   C. 30 Gy in 10 fractions
   D. Above 70 Gy.

404. **The investigation of choice for imaging of urinary tract tuberculosis is:**
   A. Plain X-ray
   B. Intravenous urography
   C. Ultrasound
   D. Computed tomography

405. **"Sunray appearance" on X-rays is suggestive of:**
   A. A chondrosarcoma
   B. A metastatic tumour in the bone
   C. An osteogenic sarcoma
   D. An Ewing's sarcoma

406. **The gold standard for the diagnosis of osteoporosis is:**
   A. Dual energy X-ray absorptiometry
   B. Single energy X-ray absorptiometry
   C. Ultrasonography
   D. Quantitative computed tomography

407. **A 33-year-old man presented with a slowly progressive swelling in the middle third of his right tibia. X-ray examination revealed multiple sharply demarcated radiolucent lesions separated by areas of dense and sclerotic bone. Microscopic examination of a biopsy specimen revealed island of epithelial cells in a fibrous stroma. Which of the following is the most probable diagnosis?**
   A. Adamantinoma
   B. Osteofibrous dysplasia
   C. Osteosarcoma
   D. Fibrous cortical defect

408. **The right lobe of the liver consists which of the following segments?**
   A. V, VI, VII and VIII
   B. IV, V, VI, VII and VIII
   C. I, V, VI, VII and VIII
   D. I, IV, V, VI, VII and VIII

409. A 25-year-old man presented with fever and cough for two months. CT chest showed bilateral upper lobe fibrosis and mediastinal enlarged necrotic nodes with peripheral rim enhancement. What is the most likely diagnosis?
    A. Sarcoidosis
    B. Tuberculosis
    C. Lymphoma
    D. Silicosis

410. Which one of the following statements is wrong regarding adult polycystic kidney disease?
    A. Kidneys are enlarged in size
    B. The presentation is unilateral
    C. Intracranial aneurysms may be associated
    D. Typically manifests in the 3rd decade

411. Angiographically, the typical "beaded" or pile of plates" appearance involving the internal carotid artery is observed in:
    A. Takayu's disease
    B. Non-specific aorto-arteritis
    C. Fibromuscular dysplasia
    D. Rendu-Osler-Weber Disease

412. Subdural hematoma most commonly results from:
    A. Rupture of intracranial aneurysm
    B. Rupture of cerebral AVM
    C. Injury to cortical bridging veins
    D. Haemophilia

413. After contrast media infection in the Radiology department, a patient develops severe hypotension, bronchospasm and cyanosis. Which one of the following drugs should be used for treatment?
    A. Atropine
    B. Aminophylline
    C. Dopamine
    D. Adrenaline

414. Which of the following usually produces osteoblastic secondaries?
    A. Carcinoma lung
    B. Carcinoma breast
    C. Carcinoma urinary bladder
    D. Carcinoma prostate

SECTION FOUR

415. A 24-year-old male, known epileptic, presented following a seizure with pain in the right shoulder region. Examination revealed that the right upper limb was adducted and internally rotated and the movements could not be performed. Which of the following is the most likely diagnosis?
    A. Posterior dislocation of shoulder.
    B. Luxatio erecta.
    C. Intrathoracic dislocation of shoulder.
    D. Subglenoid dislocation of shoulder.

416. The following features are true for Tetralogy of Fallot, except:
    A. Ventricular septal defect
    B. Right ventricular hypertrophy
    C. Atrial septal defect
    D. Pulmonary stenosis.

417. The most common retrobulbar orbital mass in adults is:
    A. Neurofibroma
    B. Meningioma
    C. Cavernous haemangioma
    D. Schwannoma

418. Expanisle type osseous metastases are characteristic of primary malignancy of:
    A. Kidney
    B. Bronchus
    C. Breast
    D. Prostate

419. Which is the objective sign of identifying pulmonary plethora in a chest radiograph?
    A. Diameter of the main pulmonary/ artery> 16mm.
    B. Diameter of the left pulmonary artery > 16mm
    C. Diameter of the descending right pulmonary artery> 16mm
    D. Diameter of the descending left pulmonary artery > 16 mm

420. The most accurate investigation for assessing ventricular function is:
    A. Multislice CT
    B. Echocardiography
    C. Nuclear scan
    D. MRI

421. The most important sign of significance of renal artery stenosis on an angiogram is:
   A. A percentage diameter stenosis> 70%
   B. Presence of collaterals
   C. A systolic pressure gradient> 20 mm Hg across the lesion
   D. Post stenotic dilatation of the renal artery

422. The MR imaging in multiple sclerosis will show lesion in:
   A. White matter
   B. Grey matter
   C. Thalamus
   D. Basal ganglia

423. The most common location of hypertensive intracranial haemorrhage is:
   A. Subarachnoid space
   B. Basal ganglia
   C. Cerebellum
   D. Brainstem

424. Which of the following causes rib- notching on the chest radiography?
   A. Bidirectional Glem shunt
   B. Modified Blalock- Taussing shunt
   C. IVC occlusion
   D. Coarctation of aorta

425. The most sensitive imaging modality to detect early renal tuberculosis is:
   A. Intravenous urography
   B. Computed tomography
   C. Ultrasound
   D. Magnetic Resonance imaging

426. All of them use non- ionizing radiation, *except*:
   A. Ultrasonography
   B. Thermography
   C. MRI
   D. Radiography

427. The most radiosensitive tumor among the following is:
   A. Bronchogenic carcinoma
   B. Carcinoma parotid
   C. Dysgerminoma
   D. Osteogenic sarcoma

428. All of the following modalites can be used for in –
situ ablation of liver secondaries, *except*:
   A. Ultrasonic waves
   B. Cryotherapy
   C. Alcohol
   D. Radiofrequency

429. All of the following radioisotopes are used as
systemic radionucleide, *except*:
   A. Phosphorus- 32
   B. Strontium – 89
   C. Iridium- 192
   D. Samarium – 153

430. Phosphorous – 32 emits:
   A. Beta particles
   B. Alfa particles
   C. Neutrons
   D. X- rays

431. Which of the following is used in the treatment of
differentiated thyroid cancer?
   A. ^{131}I
   B. ^{99m}Tc
   C. ^{32}P
   D. ^{131}I-MIBG

432. Which one of the following imaging techniques
gives maximum radiation exposure to the patient?
   A. Chest X-ray
   B. MRI
   C. CT scan
   D. Bone scan

433. Which one of the following has the maximum
ionization potential?
   A. Electron
   B. Proton
   C. Helium ion
   D. Gamma (γ)-Photon

434. Typically bilateral inferior lens subluxation of the
lens is seen in:
   A. Marfan's syndrome
   B. Homocystinuria
   C. Hyperlysinaemia
   D. Ocular trauma

435. The procedure of choice for the evaluation of an aneurysm is:
    A. Ultrasonography
    B. Computed tomography
    C. Magnetic resonance imaging
    D. Arteriography

436. The common cause of subarachnoid hemorrhage is:
    A. Arterio-venous malformation
    B. Cavenous angioma
    C. Aneurysm
    D. Hypertension

437. Spalding's sign occurs after:
    A. Birth of live foetus
    B. Death of foetus in uterus
    C. Rigor mortis of infant
    D. Cadaveric spasm.

438. Renal artery stenosis may occur in all of the following, *except*:
    A. Atherosclerosis
    B. Fibromuscular dysplasia
    C. Takayasu's arteritis
    D. Polyarteritis nodosa

439. Which one of the following congenital malformation of the fetus can be diagnosed in first trimester by ultrasound?
    A. Anencephaly
    B. Inencephaly
    C. Microcephaly
    D. Holoprosencephaly

440. Which of the following conditions is least likely to present as an acentric osteolytic lesion?
    A. Aneurysmal bone cyst
    B. Giant cell tumor
    C. Fibrous cortical defect
    D. Simple bone cyst

441. "Rugger Jersey Spine" is seen in :
    A. Fluorosis
    B. Achondroplasia
    C. Renal Osteodytrophy
    D. Marfan's Syndrome

SECTION FOUR

442. **Brown tumours are seen in:**
   A. Hyperparathyroidism
   B. Pigmented villonodular synovitis
   C. Osteomalacia
   D. Neurofibromatosis

443. **Which of the following malignant tumours is radioresistant?**
   A. Ewing's sarcoma
   B. Retinoblastoma
   C. Osteosarcoma
   D. Neuroblastoma

444. **In Radionuclide imaging the most useful radio pharmaceutical for skeletal imaging is:**
   A. Gallium 67 (^{67}Ga)
   B. Technetium-sulphur-colloid (^{99m}Tc-Sc)
   C. Technetium-99m (^{99m}Tc)
   D. Technetium-99m linked to Methylene disphos-phonate (^{99m}Tc-MDP)

445. **Which one of the following is the investigation of choice for evaluation of suspected Perthes' disease?**
   A. Plain X-ray
   B. Ultrasonography (US)
   C. Computed Tomography (CT)
   D. Magnetic Resonance Imaging (MRI)

446. **Which one of the following is the most preferred route to perform cerebral angiography?**
   A. Transfemoral route
   B. Transaxillary route
   C. Direct carotid puncture
   D. Transbrachial route

447. **Which one of the following radioisotope is *not* used as permanent implant?**
   A. Iodine-125
   B. Palladium-103
   C. Gold-198
   D. Caesium-137

448. **Which one of the following tumors shows calci-fication on CT Scan?**
   A. Ependymoma
   B. Meduloblastoma
   C. Meningioma
   D. CNS lymphoma

449. The technique employed in radiotherapy to counteract the effect of tumour motion due to breathing is known as:
   A. Arc technique
   B. Modulation
   C. Gating
   D. Shunting

450. Gamma camera in Nuclear Medicine is used for:
   A. Organ imaging
   B. Measuring the radioactivity
   C. Monitoring the surface contamination
   D. RIA

451. At t = 0 there are 6×10^{23} radioactive atoms of a substance, which decay with a disintegration constant (λ) equal to 0.01/sec. What would be the initial decay rate?
   A. 6×10^{23}
   B. 6×10^{22}
   C. 6×10^{21}
   D. 6×10^{20}

452. The most sensitive imaging modality for diagnosing ureteric stones in a patient with acute colic is:
   A. X-ray KUB region
   B. Ultrasonogram
   C. Non contrast CT scan of the abdomen
   D. Contrast enhanced CT scan of the abdomen

453. In a child, non-functioning kidney is best diagnosed by:
   A. Ultrasonography
   B. IVU
   C. DTPA renogram
   D. Creatinine clearance

454. The gold standard for the diagnosis of osteoporosis is:
   A. Dual energy X-ray absorptiometry
   B. Single energy X-ray absorptiometry
   C. Ultrasound
   D. Quantitative computed tomography

455. Which of the following ultrasound marker is associated with greatest increased risk for Trisomy 21 in fetus?
   A. Echogenic foci in heart
   B. Hyperechogenic bowel

C. Choroid plexus cysts

D. Nuchal edema

456. **Heberden's nodes are found in:**

A. PIP joints in osteoarthritis

B. DIP joints in osteoarthritis

C. PIP joints in rheumatoid arthritis

D. DIP joints in osteoarthritis

457. **Investigation of choice for detection and characterization of interstitial lung disease is:**

A. MRI

B. Chest X-ray

C. High resolution CT scan

D. Ventilation perfusion scan

458. **A 40-year-old female patient on long term steroid therapy presents with recent onset of severe pain in the right hip. Imaging modality of choice for this problem is:**

A. CT scan

B. Bone scan

C. MRI

D. Plain X-ray

459. **Which of the following techniques is the best for differentiating recurrence of brain tumour from radiation therapy induced necrosis?**

A. MRI

B. Contrast enhanced MRI

C. PET scan

D. CT scan

460. **Which of the following is the most common cause of a mixed cystic and solid suprasellar mass seen on cranial MR scan of a 10-year-old child?**

A. Pituitary Adenoma

B. Craniopharyngioma

C. Optic chiasmal glioma

D. Germinoma

461. **Which of the following is the most common cause of sclerotic skeletal metastasis in a female patient?**

A. Carcinoma breast

B. Carcinoma ovary

C. Endometrial carcinoma

D. Melanoma

462. Which of the following is the most radiosensitive tumour?
    A. Ewings tumour
    B. Hodgkin's disease
    C. Carcinoma cervix
    D. Malignant fibrous histocytoma

463. For which malignancy, intensity modulated radiotherapy (IMRT) is the most suitable?
    A. Lung
    B. Prostate
    C. Leukemias
    D. Stomach

464. In treatment of papillary carcinoma thyroid, radioiodine destroys the neoplastic cells predominantly by:
    A. X-rays
    B. β rays
    C. γ rays
    D. α particles

465. Which of the following radioactive isotopes is *not* used for brachytherapy?
    A. Iodine-125
    B. Iodine-131
    C. Cobalt-60
    D. Iridium-192

466. Solitary hypoechoic lesion of the liver without septae or debris is most likely to be:
    A. Hydatid cyst
    B. Caroli's disease
    C. Liver abscess
    D. Simple cyst

467. The posterior urethra is best visualized by:
    A. Static cystogram
    B. Retrograde urethrogram
    C. Voiding cystogram
    D. CT cystogram

468. The most definitive method of diagnosing pulmonary embolism is:
    A. Pulmonary ateriography
    B. Radioisotope perfusion pulmonary scintigraphy
    C. EKG
    D. Venography

SECTION FOUR

469. Which of the following statements is true regarding subclavian steal syndrome?
    A. Reversal of blood flow in the ipsilateral vertebral artery
    B. Reversal of blood flow in the contralateral carotid artery
    C. Reversal of blood flow in the contralateral vertebral artery
    D. Bilateral reversal of blood flow in the vertebral arteries

470. Which of the following techniques uses piezo-electric crystals?
    A. Ultrasonography
    B. NMR imaging
    C. X-ray diffraction
    D. Xeroradiography

471. In computed tomography (CT), the attenuation values are measured in Hounsfield units (HU). An attenuation value of '0 (zero) HU corresponds to:
    A. Water
    B. Air
    C. Very dense bone structures
    D. Fat

472. The EEG cabins should be completely shielded by a continuous sheet of wire mesh of copper to avoid the picking up of noise from external electromagnetic disturbances. Such a Shielding is called as:
    A. Maxwell cage
    B. Faraday cage
    C. Edison's cage
    D. Ohms cage

473. Which of the following is the incorrect statement regarding GI bleeding?
    A. The sensitivity of angiography for detecting GI bleeding is about 10-20% as compared to Nuclear Imaging
    B. Angiography can image bleeding at a rate of 0.05/0.1/min or less
    C. ^{99m}Tc-RBC scan image bleeding at rates as low 0.05-0.1 ml/min
    D. Angiography will detect bleeding only if extravasation is occurring during the injection of contrast

474. Which one of the following hepatic lesions can be diagnosed with high accuracy by using nuclear imaging?
   A. Hepatocellular carcinoma
   B. Hepatic adenoma
   C. Focal nodular hyperplasia
   D. Cholangiocarcinoma

475. Which one of the following is the earliest radiographic manifestation of childhood leukemia?
   A. Radiolucent transverse metaphyseal bands
   B. Diffuse demineralization of bones
   C. Osteoblastic lesions in skull
   D. Parenchymal pulmonary lesions on chest films

476. A 55-year-old male presents with features of obstructive jaundice. He also reports a weight loss of seven kilograms in last two months. On CT scan, the CBD is dilated till the lower end and the main pancreatic duct is also dilated. Pancreas is normal. The most likely diagnosis is:
   A. Choledocholithiasis
   B. Carcinoma Gallbladder
   C. Hilar Cholangiocarcinoma
   D. Periampullary carcinoma

477. In which of the following conditions the lead pipe appearance of the colon on a barium enema is seen?
   A. Amoebiasis
   B. Ulcerative colitis
   C. Tuberculosis of the colon
   D. Crohn's involvement of the colon

478. Patient who had an Road traffic accident presents with presents with loss of consciousness CT shows multiple spotty hemorrhages and full basal cisterns-
   A. Brain contusion
   B. Diffuse axonal injury
   C. Subdural Hematoma
   D. Multiple infarcts

479. Tumour showing dural enhancement with a tail is:
   A. Medulloblastoma
   B. Meningioma
   C. Glioma
   D. Acoustic neuroma

480. A 25-yrs-old female presented with lower limb weakness, spasticity, urinary hesitancy, mid-dorsal

intradural enhancing mass seen in MRI. What is the diagnosis?
A. Intradural lipoma
B. Meningioma
C. Dermoid cyst
D. Neuroepithelial cyst

481. A neonate presents with congestive heart failure, on examination enlarging fontanelles, bruit on auscultation, on USG shows midline hypoechoeic lesion, most likely diagnosis:
A. Malformation of vein of galen
B. Aqueduct stenosis
C. Arachnoid cyst
D. Medulloblastoma.

482. Best investigation for temporal bone fracture is:
A. CT   B. MRI
C. X-RAY   D. Ultrasound

483. Spongy mass with sunburst calcification in center seen in CT is seen in:
A. Mucinous cystadenoma CA
B. Serous Cystadenoca
C. Somatostationoma
D. Adenocarcinoma pancreas

484. Which of the following is not sensitive to Radio-therapy?
A. Ewings sarcoma
B. Osteosarcoma
C. Wilms'
D. Neuroblastoma

485. 60 year old man with sensorineural deafness and bony abnormality in left leg has S.Ca2+-9.5 and alkaline phosphate 440mu/l skeletal survey shows ivory vertebra and cotton wool spots on skull most probable diagnosis:
A. Paget's disease
B. Osteosclerotic metastasis
C. Osteoporosis
D. Fibrous dysplasia

486. Bohler's angle is seen in:
A. Calcaneum
B. Talus
C. Navicular
D. Cuboid

487. **Not seen in OSTEOPETROSIS?**
    A. Pancytopenia
    B. Delayed healing of fractures
    C. Compression of cranial nerve
    D. Osteomyelitis of mandible

488. **Material used in vertebroplasty?**
    A. Polymethyl methacrylate
    B. IsoMethyl Methacrylate
    C. Isoethyl Methacrylayte
    D. Silicon

489. **Gold standard test for diagnosis of acoustic neuroma?**
    A. CT with contrast
    B. MRI with contrast
    C. CT without contrast
    D. Angiography

490. **Loss of cardiac silhoutee is seen in pathology of?**
    A. Rt. Middle lobe
    B. Rt. Lower lobe
    C. Rt. Atria
    D. Rt. Ventricle

491. **Snowman's appearance is seen in which cardiac pathology?**
    A. TOF
    B. Fallot's tetralogy
    C. Corrected TGA
    D. TAPVC

492. **Egg on side appearance is seen in?**
    A. Ebstein anomaly
    B. Uncorrected TGA
    C. Tricuspid atresia
    D. Tetralogy of fallot

493. **The most chemoresistant tumor amongst the following?**
    A. Synovial sarcoma
    B. Malignant fibrous histiocytoma
    C. Osteosarcoma
    D. Clear cell sarcoma

494. **Which of this is not a sign of increased ICT?**
    A. Copper beaten appearance

B. Erosion of dorsum sella

C. Ballooning of sella

D. Sutural diastasis

495. Hair on end appearance is seen in?

A. Thalassemia

B. Scurvy

C. Rickets

D. Sickle cell disease

496. PACS in medical imaging stands for?

A. Portal archiving common system

B. Planning archiving communication scheme

C. Picture archiving communication system*

D. Photo archiving computerised system

497. Extensive involvement of deep white matter with hyperintense thalamic lesion on non-contrast CT scan of the brain is seen in:

A. Krabbe's disease

B. Alexander disease

C. Metrachromatic Leukodystrophy

D. Cannavan's disease

498. Most diagnostic of pulmonary embolism in a high-risk case is:

A. Multidetector CT angiography

B. Catheter angiography

C. D-dimer

D. Ventilation perfusion scan

499. Hamptoms Hump is seen in:

A. Pulmonary embolism

B. Tuberculosis

C. Bronchogenic Ca

D. Pneumonia

500. A child presents with multiple vertebral anomalies and a posterior mediastinal mass. Likely diagnosis is:

A. Neuroenteric cyst

B. Meningomyelocele

C. Bronchogenic cyst

D. Neuroblastoma

501. Which of the following statements about acute Cholecystitis is true?

A. It usually occurs due to obstruction at the neck of gall bladder

B. On HIDA scan, gall bladder is not visualized

C. Immediate cholecystectomy can never be done

D. Analgesics and intravenous fluids are the best treatment

502. **True about umbilical artery Doppler is:**

A. Changes in the flow velocity waveforms of umbilical artery may be important in the management of high-risk pregnancies*

B. Absence of end-diastolic flow is normal at term

C. Maternal smoking decreases S/D ratio

D. Increased diastolic flow indicates worse prognosis

503. **Which radionuclide is best suited for measurement of GFR?**

A. DTPA

B. DMSA

C. Orthoiodohippurate

D. EDTA

504. **Best view for visualizing C1 and C2 vertebrae is:**

A. AP

B. Lateral

C. Odontoid

D. Oblique

505. **Fraying of anterior ends of ribs is seen in:**

A. Scurvy

B. Rickets

C. Down syndrome

D. Osteoporosis

506. **Earliest sign of pulmonary venus hypertension on chest radiograph is:**

A. Pleural effusion

B. Kerley B lines

C. Cephalization of veins

D. Kerley a lines

507. **Earliest sign of left atrial hypertrophy is:**

A. Posterior displacement of esophagus

B. Widening of carinal angle

SECTION FOUR

C. Upward displacement of left bronchus

D. Double contour of right border of heart

508. **Most sensitive phase to radiotherapy is:**

A. G1

B. S

C. G2M

D. M

509. **Photoelectric effect is based on the principle that a photon:**

A. Interacts with electrons in outermost orbit

B. Interacts with electrons in the inner shells (K Shell)

C. Interacts with nucleus

D. Does not interact with the atom

510. **Which of the following features is not seen ileo-caecal tuberculosis?**

A. Pulled up caecum

B. Apple core appearance

C. Obliteration of angle between ileum and caecum

D. Narrowing of distal end of caecum

511. **Characteristic radiographic appearance of aortitis is:**

A. Calcification of ascending aorta

B. Calcification of desecending aorta

C. Dilation of arch of aorta

D. Enlargement of left atrium

512. **Radicontrast reactions are mostly:**

A. Anaphylactoid reactions

B. IgE-Mediated reactions

C. Delayed hypersensitivity reactions

D. Immune complex mediated reactions

513. **Planned radiation volume is:**

A. Depends on 90% of tumour size

B. Less than targeted radiation volume

C. More than targeted radiation volume

D. Equal to targeted radiation volume

514. **Conformation radiotherapy uses:**

A. Multileaf collimator

B. Single leaf collimator

C. Cone

D. Cylinder

515. **Floating teeth is seen in:**
     A. Hyperparathyroidism
     B. Hypoparathyroidism
     C. Rickets
     D. Scurvy

516. **Bare orbit sign is seen in:**
     A. NF I
     B. NF II
     C. Sturge weber syndrome
     D. Tuberous sclerosis

517. **In Tuberous sclerosis all are seen except:**
     A. Subependymal nodules
     B. Tubers
     C. Giant cell Astrocytoma
     D. Ependymoma

518. **Inferior rib notching is seen in all *except*:**
     A. Blalock taussig shunt operation
     B. Aortic interruption
     C. Waterson cooley's shunt
     D. Pulmonary stenosis with vsd

519. **Radioactive element not used nowadays in medical practice:**
     A. Radium 226
     B. Co60
     C. Cs 137
     D. Iridium 192

520. **Investigation of choice for vascular ring around airway:**
     A. PET
     B. CT
     C. MRI
     D. Catheter directed angiography

521. **Radiation induced necrosis can be diagnosed by:**
     A. PET
     B. MRI
     C. Biopsy
     D. CT

522. **On barium swallow posterior indentation is seen due to:**

A. Left atrium

B. Aortic knuckle

C. Aberrant right subclavian

D. Sling of pulmonary artery

523. **Investigation of choice for a lesion of temporal bone:**

A. CT

B. MRI

C. USG

D. Plain X-ray

524. **Characteristic radiological feature of fibrous dysplasia**

A. Thickened bone matrix

B. Cortical erosion

C. Ground glass appearance

D. Bone enlargement

525. **Bohler's angle is seen in:**

A. Calcaneum

B. Talus

C. Navicular

D. Cuboid

526. **What is the full form of dicom?**

A. Digital imaging and communications in medicine

B. Direct imaging and colors in medicine

C. Dependent interconnectivity in medicine

D. Digital information and connectivity in medicine

527. **Nephrogenic systemic fibrosis is associated with:**

A. Gadolinium administration in CRF

B. Genetic disease with selenium deficiency

C. Chromium toxicity

D. HIV associated

528. **"Tear drop sign" is seen on waters view in:**

A. Blow out fracture

B. Maxillary mucocele

C. Nasolacrimal duct blockage

D. Fibrous dysplasia

529. **Which cancer is predisposed by radon exposure?**

A. Lung

B. Cervix

C. Oral cavity

D. Bladder

530. **Current gold standard to detect ductal carcinoma in situ breast is:**

   A. Mammography

   B. MRI

   C. USG

   D. CT/PET

531. **Isotope used for myocardial perfusion pet is:**

   A. Rubidium 82

   B. FDG

   C. Thymidine

532. **Half life f-18 is:**

   A. 110 min

   B. 90 min

   C. 6 hours

   D. 13 days

533. **Delta sign on NCCT head is seen in:**

   A. Infarct

   B. Superior saggital sinus thrombosis

   C. SAH

   D. EDH

ANSWERS

1	D	(Page 22)	2	B	(Page 53)
3	B	(Page 60)	4	A	(Page 54)
5	A	(Page 80)	6	C	(Page 11)
7	A	(Page 34)	8	A	(Page 70)
9	A	(Page 72)	10	A	(Page 54)
11	D	(Page 29)	12	A	(Page 27)
13	D	(Page 87)	14	C	(Page 61)
15	B	(Page 70)	16	A	(Page 59)
17	B	(Page 57)	18	B	(Page 62)
19	C	(Page 22)	20	D	(Page 60)
21	A	(Page 68)	22	C	(Page 109)
23	B	(Page 54)	24	B	(Page 111)
25	D	(Page 4)	26	A	(Page 65)
27	D	(Page 80)	28	C	(Page 7)
29	A	(Page 63)	30	C	(Page 1)
31	D	(Page 12)	32	C	(Page 15)
33	A	(Page 14)	34	D	(Page 13)
35	C	(Page 80)	36	C	(Page 12)
37	D	(Page 85)	38	B	(Page 106)
39	C	(Page 7)	40	D	(Page 30)
41	D	(Page 1)	42	C	(Page 14)
43	D	(Page 98)	44	A	(Page 114)
45	A		46	B	(Page 98)
47	A, B	(Page 30)	48	D	(Page 36)
49	D	(Page 14)	50	A	(Page 13)
51	B	(Page 22)	52	B	(Page 69)
53	B	(Page 111)	54	A	(Page 34)
55	C	(Page 93)	56	D	(Page 31)
57	A	(Page 13)	58	B	(Page 22)
59	B	(Page 111)	60	D	(Page 85)
61	B	(Page 54)	62	E	(Page 67)
63	A	(Page 51)	64	C	(Page 11)
65	A	(Page 61)	66	B	(Page 2)
67	A	(Page 2)	68	E	(Page 111)
69	A	(Page 70)	70	B	(Page 24)
71	A	(Page 80)	72	C	(Page 59)
73	D	(Page 47)	74	A	(Page 96)

SECTION FOUR

75	C	*(Page 58)*	76	A	*(Page 25)*
77	B	*(Page 80)*	78	C	*(Page 72)*
79	A	*(Page 6)*	80	B	*(Page 74)*
81	C	*(Page 74)*	82	B	*(Page 9)*
83	B	*(Page 74)*	84	C	*(Page 22)*
85	A	*(Page 111)*	86	C	*(Page 74)*
87	A	*(Page 66)*	88	A	*(Page 65)*
89	D	*(Page 14)*	90	C	*(Page 77)*
91	B	*(Page 33)*	92	A	*(Page 30)*
93	C	*(Page 94)*	94	A	*(Page 97)*
95	A	*(Page 24)*	96	B	*(Page 57)*
97	C	*(Page 7)*	98	B	*(Page 12)*
99	B	*(Page 7)*	100	D	*(Page 30)*
101	B	*(Page 49)*	102	A	*(Page 26)*
103	B	*(Page 28)*	104	A	
105	A	*(Page 104)*	106	A	*(Page 1)*
107	D	*(Page 21)*	108	A	*(Page 35)*
109	B	*(Page 114)*	110	D	
111	A	*(Page 3)*	112	C	*(Page 43)*
113	D	*(Page 90)*	114	A	*(Page 90)*
115	C	*(Page 32)*	116	B	*(Page 7)*
117	A,C	*(Page 7)*	118	D	*(Page 25)*
119	A	*(Page 21)*	120	D	*(Page 93)*
121	C	*(Page 35)*	122	B	*(Page 7)*
123	A	*(Page 35)*	124	A	*(Page 114)*
125	C	*(Page 6)*	126	D	*(Page 70)*
127	A	*(Page 39)*	128	C	*(Page 134)*
129	A	*(Page 108)*	130	D	
131	A	*(Page 7)*	132	D	*(Page 14)*
133	D	*(Page 34)*	134	B	*(Page 6)*
135	B	*(Page 100)*	136	B	
137	B	*(Page 7)*	138	B	*(Page 15)*
139	C	*(Page 10)*	140	B	
141	A	*(Page 69)*	142	C	*(Page 22)*
143	C	*(Page 114)*	144	A	*(Page 4)*
145	A	*(Page 10)*	146	A	*(Page 74)*
147	B	*(Page 84)*	148	B	*(Page 55)*
149	A	*(Page 93)*	150	C	*(Page 27)*
151	A	*(Page 110)*	152	C	*(Page 7)*
153	A	*(Page 5)*	154	C	*(Page 5)*
155	D	*(Page 18)*	156	B	*(Page 17)*
157	E	*(Page 19)*	158	E	*(Page 15)*

159	D	*(Page 70)*	160	A	*(Page 13)*
161	E	*(Page 120)*	162	D	*(Page 120, 121)*
163	D	*(Page 85)*	164	C	*(Page 111)*
165	D	*(Page 84)*	166	D	*(Page 44)*
167	C	*(Page 22)*	168	D	*(Page 36)*
169	A	*(Page 123)*	170	A	*(Page 19)*
171	C	*(Page 7)*	172	B	*(Page 5)*
173	B	*(Page 70)*	174	B	*(Page 118)*
175	A	*(Page 14)*	176	D	*(Page 96)*
177	B	*(Page 108)*	178	B	*(Page 13)*
179	A	*(Page 110)*	180	A,C	*(Page 111)*
181	A,B,C	*(Page 39)*	182	A,D	*(Page 69)*
183	C	*(Page 13)*	184	A	
185	D	*(Page 39)*	186	D	*(Page 17)*
187	B	*(Page 55)*	188	B	*(Page 10)*
189	C	*(Page 100)*	190	A	*(Page 1)*
191	A	*(Page 84)*	192	A	*(Page 108)*
193	A	*(Page 26)*	194	C	*(Page 24)*
195	C	*(Page 80)*	196	A	*(Page 69)*
197	C	*(Page 32)*	198	D	*(Page 4)*
199	A	*(Page 4)*	200	B	*(Page 2)*
201	A		202	A	*(Page 32)*
203	B	*(Page 22)*	204	A	*(Page 51)*
205	C		206	A	*(Page 54)*
207	A	*(Page 31)*	208	B	*(Page 44)*
209	B	*(Page 2)*	210	D	*(Page 4)*
211	B		212	B	*(Page 52)*
213	A		214	A,C	
215	C	*(Page 72)*	216	C	*(Page 2)*
217	A	*(Page 47)*	218	A	*(Page 7)*
219	A	*(Page 30)*	220	A	*(Page 34)*
221	A	*(Page 4)*	222	A	*(Page 94)*
223	D	*(Page 84)*	224	E	*(Page 44)*
225	C	*(Page 109)*	226	C	
227	A,B		228	D	
229	A	*(Page 22)*	230	B	
231	C	*(Page 22)*	232	A	*(Page 7)*
233	B	*(Page 59)*	234	D	*(Page 46)*
235	B	*(Page 64)*	236	A	*(Page 16)*
237	A,C	*(Page 30)*	238	C	*(Page 39)*
239	B	*(Page 115)*	240	A,C	*(Page 235)*

241	C		242	A	(Page 19)
243	A	(Page 111)	244	A	(Page 57)
245	C	(Page 34)	246	B	(Page 24)
247	A		248	D	(Page 7)
249	A,D	(Page 44)	250	D	(Page 12)
251	B	(Page 111)	252	A	(Page 2)
253	B	(Page 74)	254	A	(Page 45)
255	C	(Page 27)	256	B	(Page 14)
257	A	(Page 19)	258	A	(Page 90)
259	A	(Page 90)	260	B	(Page 17)
261	A	(Page 39)	262	A	(Page 74)
263	D		264	D	
265	B		266	D	(Page 126)
267	D	(Page 64)	268	D	(Page 110)
269	D	(Page 110)	270	B	
271	D	(Page 32)	272	C	(Page 24)
273	A	(Page 10)	274	C	(Page 7)
275	B	(Page 15)	276	D	(Page 7)
277	D		278	C	(Page 22)
279	C		280	B	(Page 74)
281	B,E	(Page 35)	282	B	(Page 16)
283	B	(Page 90)	284	A	(Page 6)
285	D		286	D	(Page 16)
287	A	(Page 113)	288	A	
289	B	(Page 95)	290	A	(Page 13)
291	D	(Page 34)	292	A	
293	E	(Page 44)	294	A	
295	B	(Page 39)	296	A	(Page 34)
297	C		298	A	(Page 87)
299	A		300	C	(Page 14)
301	C	(Page 78)	302	C	(Page 109)
303	A		304	C	(Page 102)
305	C	(Page 92)	306	A	(Page 90)
307	C	(Page 81)	308	B	
309	C	(Page 62)	310	B	(Page 3)
311	D	(Page 26)	312	A	
313	C	(Page 46)	314	D	(Page 33)
315	A	(Page 74)	316	C	(Page 6)
317	C	(Page 36)	318	A	(Page 35)
319	C	(Page 39)	320	B	(Page 13)
321	B	(Page 8)	322	C	(Page 21)

SECTION FOUR

323	A	*(Page 130)*	324	D	
325	A	*(Page 110)*	326	D	*(Page 21)*
327	B	*(Page 21)*	328	A	
329	B		330	A	*(Page 16)*
331	A	*(Page 14)*	332	A	*(Page 114)*
333	A	*(Page 44)*	334	C	*(Page 32)*
335	D		336	A	*(Page 36)*
337	A		338	B	*(Page 7)*
339	D	*(Page 19)*	340	A	*(Page 54)*
341	D	*(Page 36)*	342	D	*(Page 22)*
343	D		344	A	
345	A	*(Page 95)*	346	A	*(Page 39)*
347	B	*(Page 94)*	348	D	*(Page 19)*
349	A	*(Page 65)*	350	D	
351	A	*(Page 80)*	352	D	*(Page 1)*
353	D	*(Page 30)*	354	C	*(Page 31)*
355	C	*(Page 90)*	356	A	*(Page 14)*
357	B	*(Page 5)*	358	B	*(Page 80)*
359	C		360	B	
361	A	*(Page 14)*	362	D	*(Page 5)*
363	A	*(Page 48)*	364	D	*(Page 39)*
365	B		366	A	*(Page 97)*
367	A		368	C	
369	A	*(Page 73)*	370	D	*(Page 59)*
371	B		372	A	*(Page 69)*
373	A	*(Page 18)*	374	D	
375	B	*(Page 85)*	376	A	*(Page 89)*
377	B	*(Page 109)*	378	A	*(Page 34)*
379	A	*(Page 134)*	380	C	*(Page 109)*
381	D	*(Page 14)*	382	B	*(Page 22)*
383	B	*(Page 54)*	384	B	*(Page 74)*
385	B	*(Page 27)*	386	D	*(Page 44)*
387	A	*(Page 33)*	388	D	*(Page 85)*
389	B		390	C	*(Page 102)*
391	C	*(Page 133)*	392	B	*(Page 27)*
393	D	*(Page 111)*	394	B	*(Page 11)*
395	B	*(Page 85)*	396	D	*(Page 85)*
397	B	*(Page 22)*	398	B	*(Page 46)*
399	D	*(Page 32)*	400	B	*(Page 48)*
401	B	*(Page 73)*	402	A	*(Page 67)*
403	C	*(Page 118)*	404	B	*(Page 79)*

405	C	*(Page 59)*	**406**	A	*(Page 54)*
407	A	*(Page 61)*	**408**	A	*(Page 75)*
409	B	*(Page 27)*	**410**	B	*(Page 80)*
411	C	*(Page 82)*	**412**	C	*(Page 6)*
413	D	*(Page 11)*	**414**	D	*(Page 63)*
415	A	*(Page 64)*	**416**	C	*(Page 44)*
417	C	*(Page 94)*	**418**	A	*(Page 63)*
419	C	*(Page 41)*	**420**	D	*(Page 17)*
421	B	*(Page 83)*	**422**	A	*(Page 93)*
423	B		**424**	D	*(Page 44)*
425	A	*(Page 79)*	**426**	D	*(Page 7)*
427	C	*(Page 109)*	**428**	C	*(Page 77)*
429	C	*(Page 122)*	**430**	A	*(Page 122)*
431	A	*(Page 18)*	**432**	D	*(Page 23)*
433	C	*(Page 102)*	**434**	B	
435	D		**436**	C	*(Page 89)*
437	B	*(Page 95)*	**438**	D	*(Page 82-83)*
439	A	*(Page 95)*	**440**	D	*(Page 61)*
441	C	*(Page 54)*	**442**	A	*(Page 53)*
443	C	*(Page 109)*	**444**	D	*(Page 19)*
445	D	*(Page 56)*	**446**	A	*(Page 14)*
447	D	*(Page 114)*	**448**	C	*(Page 86)*
449	C	*(Page 112)*	**450**	B	*(Page 16)*
451	C	*(Page 101)*	**452**	C	*(Page 79)*
453	C	*(Page 16)*	**454**	A	*(Page 54)*
455	D	*(Page 49)*	**456**	B	*(Page 58)*
457	C	*(Page 5)*	**458**	C	*(Page 56)*
459	C	*(Page 20)*	**460**	B	*(Page 85)*
461	A	*(Page 63)*	**462**	B	*(Page 108)*
463	B	*(Page 121)*	**464**	B	*(Page 18)*
465	B	*(Page 114)*	**466**	D	*(Page 75)*
467	C	*(Page 14)*	**468**	A	*(Page 34)*
469	A	*(Page 89)*	**470**	A	*(Page 7)*
471	A	*(Page 6)*	**472**	B	*(Page 9)*
473	B	*(Page 18)*	**474**	C	*(Page 19)*
475	A	*(Page 56)*	**476**	D	*(Page 75)*
477	B	*(Page 70)*	**478**	B	*(Page 235)*
479	B	*(Page 235)*	**480**	B	*(Page 235)*
481	A	*(Page 235)*	**482**	A	*(Page 10)*

SECTION FOUR

483	B	*(Page 235)*	484	B	*(Page 109)*
485	A	*(Page 56)*	486	A	*(Page 235)*
487	B		488	A	*(Page 245)*
489	B		490	A	*(Page 26)*
491	D	*(Page 44)*	492	B	*(Page 45)*
493	B	*(Page 109)*	494	C	*(Page 85)*
495	A	*(Page 55)*	496	C	*(Page 241)*
497	A	*(Page 244)*	498	A	*(Page 245)*
499	A	*(Page 33)*	500	A	*(Page 41)*
501	B	*(Page 13)*	502	A	*(Page 246)*
503	A	*(Page 16)*	504	C	
505	B	*(Page 54)*	506	C	*(Page 32)*
507	D	*(Page 39)*	508	C	*(Page 21)*
509	B		510	B	*(Page 69)*
511	A		512	A	*(Page 11)*
613	C		514	A	
515	A		516	A	
517	D		518	C	*(Page 44)*
519	A	*(Page 114)*	520	B	*(Page 247)*
521	A	*(Page 20)*	522	C	*(Page 247)*
523	A		524	C	*(Page 62)*
525	A	*(Page 241)*	526	A	*(Page 241)*
527	A	*(Page 242)*	528	A	
529	A		530	B	
531	A	*(Page 20)*	532	A	*(Page 20)*
533	B	*(Page 248)*			

Section 5
Radiological Quiz

SPOT THE DIAGNOSIS

CHEST

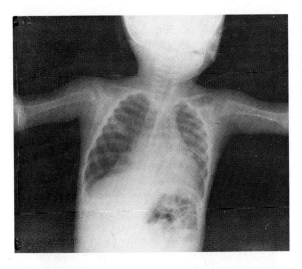

Fig. 5.1

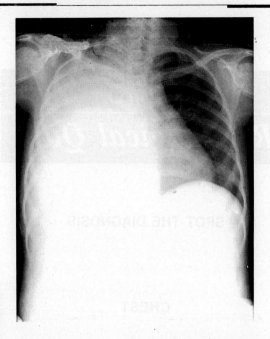

Fig. 5.2

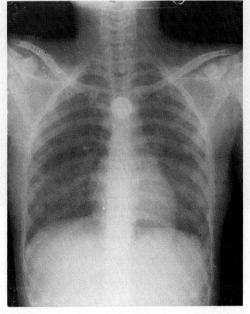

Fig. 5.3

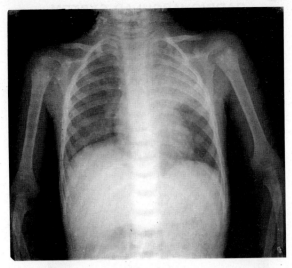

Fig. 5.4

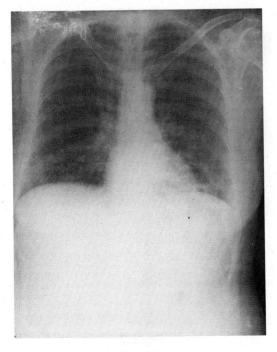

Fig. 5.5

CARDIOVASCULAR SYSTEM

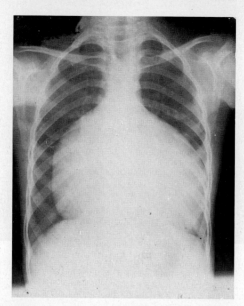

Fig. 5.6

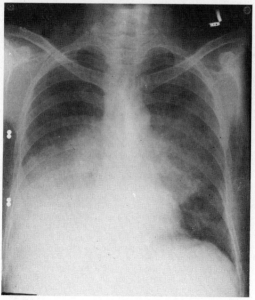

Fig. 5.7

SKELETAL SYSTEM

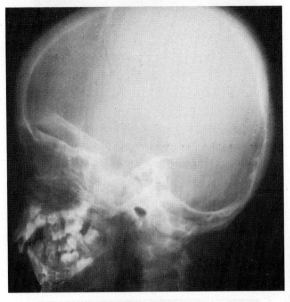

Fig. 5.8

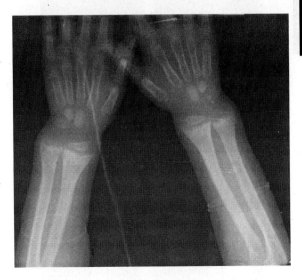

Fig. 5.9

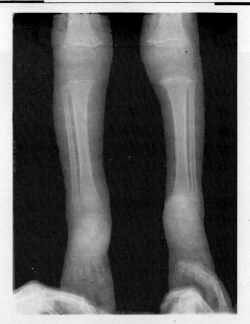

Fig. 5.10

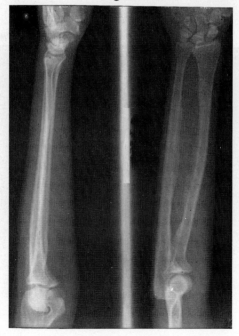

Fig. 5.11

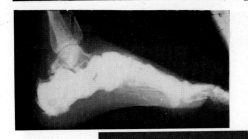

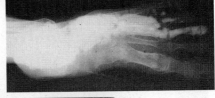

Fig. 5.12

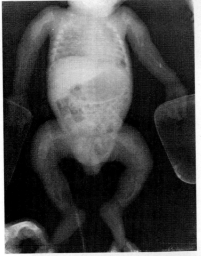

Fig. 5.13

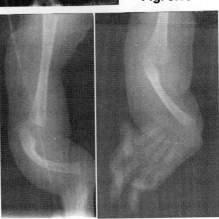

Fig. 5.14

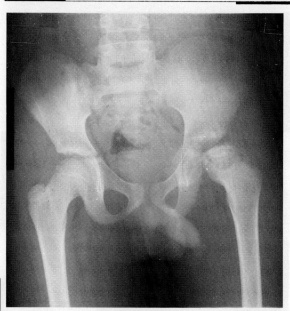

Fig. 5.15

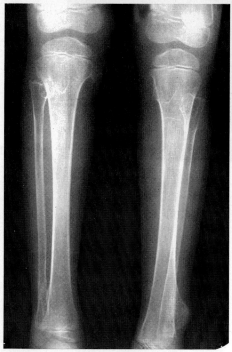

Fig. 5.16

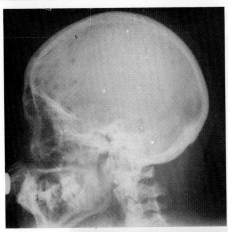

Fig. 5.17

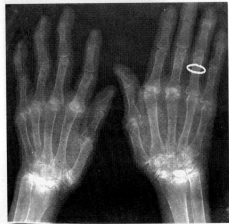

Fig. 5.18

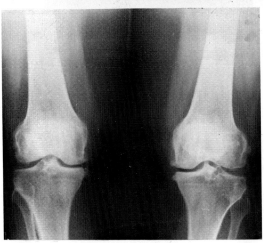

Fig. 5.19

GASTROINTESTINAL TRACT

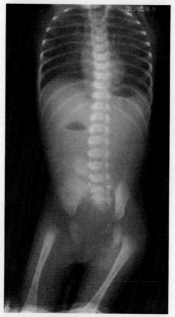

Fig. 5.20

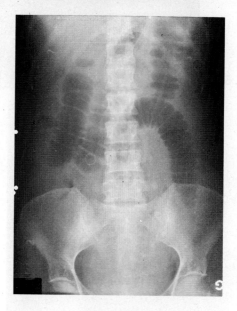

Fig. 5.21

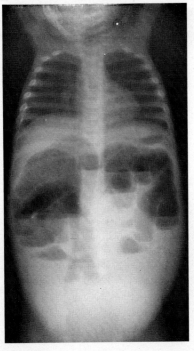

Fig. 5.22

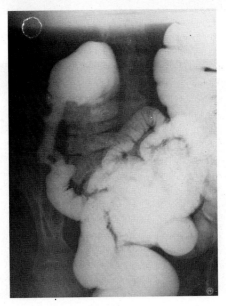

Fig. 5.23

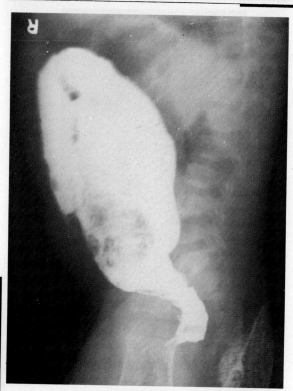

Fig. 5.24

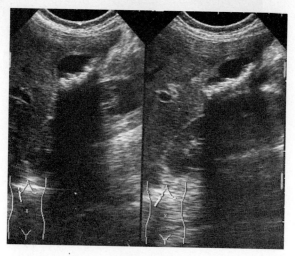

Fig. 5.25

URINARY TRACT

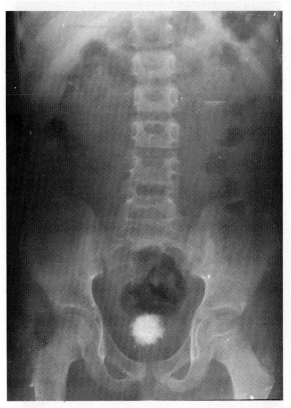

Fig. 5.26

CENTRAL NERVOUS SYSTEM

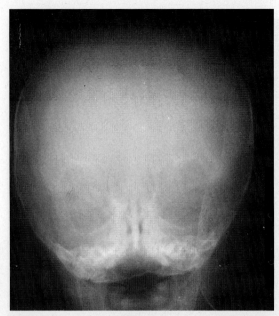

Fig. 5.27

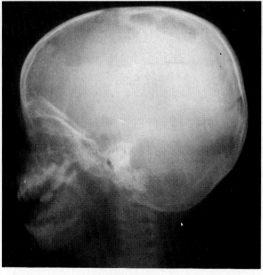

Fig. 5.28

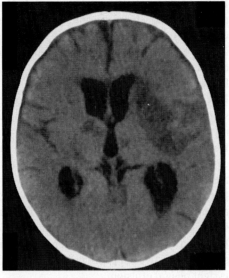

Fig. 5.29

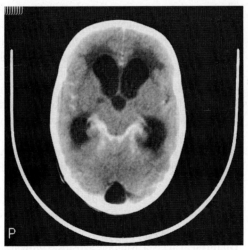

Fig. 5.30

ANSWERS

1. **Right sided pneumothorax.** There is evidence of right pneumothorax with underlying lung collapse and mediastinal shift.
2. **Massive right pleural effusion.** Other causes of opaque right hemothorax.
3. Foreign body esophagus.
4. **Left upper zone consolidation.** Homogenous opacity seen in LUZ with evidence of air bronchogram and no tracheal/mediastinal shift.
5. **Left retrocardiac cystic bronchiectasis.** Multiple cystic lucencies seen in the left retrocardiac region; the "bunch of grapes" appearance.
6. **Pericardial effusion.** The classic "money bag" heart appearance with relatively clear lung fields and no specific cardiac chamber enlargement.
7. **Pulmonary edema.** Bat wing appearance on CXR suggestive of alveolar pulmonary edema. Also noted is right pleural effusion.
8. **Hemolytic anemia.** There is evidence of diploic widening, with hair-on-end or crew-cut appearance. There is relative sparing of occipital bone.
9. **Rickets.** There is widening of the growth plate with cupping, splaying and fraying of metaphysis.
10. **Scurvy.** Evidence of a metaphyseal dense band "white line of frenkel" and a sclerotic rim to epiphysis is noted "wimberger sign"
11. **Fluorosis.** Ossification of interosseous membrane.
12. **Melorheostosis.** The classic "molten candle wax" appearance in a sclerotomal distribution.
13. **Osteogenesis imperfecta.** Multiple diaphyseal fractures. D/D battered baby in which fractures are metaphyseal.
14. **Absent radius.** Associated disorders.
15. **Perthe's disease.** Left femoral capital epiphysis is flattened and sclerotic.
16. **Diaphyseal aclasia.** Multiple exostoses growing away from the joint are noted.
17. **Multiple myeloma.** Multiple lytic lesions in the skull "rain drop appearance" D/D-lytic metastasis.
18. **Rheumatoid arthritis.** Evidence of decreased joint spaces, with erosions, osteoporosis and deformities.

19. **Osteoarthritis.** Osteophytic changes seen in bilateral tibiofemoral articular surfaces.

20. **Duodenal atresia.** "Double bubble appearance". Also seen in annular pancreas.

21. **Supine film; small bowel obstruction.** Dilated centrally placed bowel loops with valvule connvinates.

22. **Erect film; intestinal obstruction.** Multiple air-fluid levels noted.

23. **Ileocaecal Kochs.** Contracted caecum and ascending colon with stricture terminal ileum.

24. **Hirschsprung's disease.** Transition zone between normal caliber rectum and distended, fecal loaded sigmoid colon.

25. **Gall stones.** Gall stones on USG appear echogenic with acoustic shadowing.

26. **Vesical calculus.** 90% of the urinary calculi are radiopaque while only 10% of gallstones are radiopaque.

27. **Hydrocephalus.** Large head with sutural diastasis.

28. **Histiocytosis.** The classic "geographic skull" appearance.

29. **Infarcts.** Hypodense areas noted in region of bilateral internal capsules and basal ganglia region.

30. **Tubercular meningitis.** There is evidence of obliteration of basal cisterns with enhancing basal exudates and communicating hydrocephalus.

Section 6

Some Additional Mnemonics in Radiology

Transverse Lucent Metaphyseal Lines

Mnemonic: **"Lining"**
  Leukemia
  Illness, systemic (rickets, scurvy)
  Normal variant
  Infection, transplacental (congenital syphilis)
  Neuroblastoma metastases
  Growth lines

Frayed Metaphyses

Mnemonic: **"Charms"**
  Congenital infections (rubella, syphilis)
  Hypophosphatasia
  Achondroplasia
  Rickets
  Metaphyseal dysostosis
  Scurvy

Tumor Position in Longitudinal Plane

A. Epiphyseal lesion

Mnemonic: **"Caggie"**
  Chondroblastoma
  Aneurysmal bone cyst
  Giant cell tumor
  Geode
  Infection
  Eosinophilic Granuloma
(After 40 years of age throw out **"CEA"** and inset
metastases/myeloma)
B. Metaphyseal lesion
  1. Nonossifying fibroma (close to growth plate)
  2. Chondromyxoid fibroma (abutting growth plate)

3. Solitary bone cyst
4. Osteochondroma
5. Brodie abscess
6. Osteogenic sarcoma, chondrosarcoma

C. Diaphyseal Lesion

Mnemonic: **"Female"**
Fibrous dysplasia
Eosinophilic granuloma
Metastasis
Adamantinoma
Leukemia, lymphoma
Ewing sarcoma

Sarcomas by Age:

Mnemonic: **"Every Other Runner Feels Crampy Pain On Moving"**

Ewing sarcoma	0-10 years
Osteogenic sarcoma	10-30 years
Reticulum cell sarcoma	20-40 years
Fibrosarcoma	20-40 years
Chondrosarcoma	40-50 years
Parosteal sarcoma	40-50 years
Osteosarcoma	60-70 years
Metastases	60-70 years

Round Cell Tumours:
Arise in midshaft
Osteolytic lesion
Reactive new bone formation
No tumor new bone

Mnemonic: **"Lemon"**
Leukemia, Lymphoma
Ewing sarcoma, Eosinophilic Granuloma
Multiple myeloma
Osteomyelitis
Neuroblastoma

Malignancy with soft-tissue involvement

Mnemonic: **"My Mother Eats Chocolate Fudge Often"**
Metastasis
Myeloma
Ewing sarcoma
Chondrosarcoma
Fibrosarcoma
Osteosarcoma

Erlenmeyer Flask Deformity
= expansion of distal end of long bones, usually femur

Mnemonic: **"TOP DOG"**

    Thalassemia
    Osteopetrosis
    Pyle disease
    Diaphyseal aclasis
    Ollier disease
    Gaucher disease

Expansile Rib Lesion

Mnemonic: **"O Feel The Clamp"**

    Osteochondroma (25% of all benign rib tumors)
    Fibrous dysplasia
    Eosinophilic granuloma
    Enchondroma (7% of all benign rib tumors)
    Lymphoma/Leukemia
    Tuberculosis
    Hematopoiesis
    Ewing sarcoma
    Chondromyxoid fibroma
    Lymphangiomatosis
    Aneurysmal bone cyst
    Metastases
    Plasmacytoma

Metacarpal Sign

= relative shortening of 4th + 5th metacarpals

Mnemonic: **"Ping Pong Is Tough To Teach"**

    Pseudohypoparathyroidism
    Pseudopseudohypoparathyroidism
    Idiopathic
    Trauma
    Turner syndrome
    Trisomy 13-18

Heel Pad Thickening

= heel pad thickening > 25 mm (normal < 21 mm)

Mnemonic: **"MAD COP"**

    Myxedema
    Acromegaly
    Dilantin therapy
    Callus
    Obesity
    Peripheral edema

Occurrence of Bone Centers at Elbow

Mnemonic: **"CRITOE"**

Capitellum	1 year	(3-6 months)
Radial head	4 years	(3-6 years)

Internal humeral epicondyle	7 years	(5-7 years, last to fuse)
Trochlea	10 years	(9-10 years)
Olecranon	10 years	(6-10 years)
External humeral epicondyle	11 years	(9-13 years)

Carpal Bones

Mnemonic: **"Some Lovers Try Positions That They Can't Handle"**

Proximal row	*Distal row*
Scaphoid	Trapezium
Lunate	Trapezoid
Triquetrum	Capitate
Pisiform	Hamate

Avascular Necrosis

Mnemonic: **"Plastic Rags"**
   Pancreatitis, Pregnancy
   Legg-Perthes disease, Lupus erythematosus
   Alcoholism, Atherosclerosis
   Steroids
   Trauma (femoral neck fracture, hip dislocation)
   Idiopathic (Legg-Perthes disease), Infection
   Caisson disease, collagen disease (SLE)
   Rheumatoid arthritis, Radiation treatment
   Amyloid
   Gaucher disease
   Sickle cell disease

Mnemonic: **"Give Infarcts"**
   Gaucher disease
   Idiopathic (Legg-Calv,-Perthes, K"hler, Chanler)
   Vasculitis (SLE, polyarteritis nodosa, rheumatoid arthritis)
   Environmental (frostbite, thermal injury)
   Irradiation
   Neoplasia (-assocaited coagulopathy)
   Fat (prolonged corticosteroid use increases marrow)
   Alcoholism
   Renal failure + dialysis
   Caisson disease
   Trauma (femoral neck fracture, hip dislocation
   Sickle cell disease

Tumours Causing Skeletal Metastasis

Mnemonic: **"Several Kinds of Horribly Nasty Tumors Leap Promptly to Bone"**
   Sarcoma, Squamous cell carcinoma
   Kidney tumor

Ovarian cancer
Hodgkin disese
Neuroblastoma
Testicular cancer
Lung cancer
Prostate cancer
Thyroid cancer
Breast cancer

Osteoblastic Bone Metastases

Mnemonic: **"4 Bees Lick Pollen"**
Brain (medulloblastoma)
Bronchus
Breast
Bowel (especially carcinoid)
Bladder
Lymphoma
Prostate

Neuropathic joints

Mnemonic: **"DS6"**
Diabetes
Syphilis   Spina bifida
Steroids   Syringomyelia
Spinal cord injury   Scleroderma

Causes of Early Osteoarthritis

Mnemonic: **"Early Osteo Arthritis"**
Epiphyseal dysplasia, multiple
Ochronosis
Acromegaly

Rickets

Mnemonic: **"Rickets"**
Reaction of periosteum may occur
Indistinct cortex
Coarse trabeculation
Knees + wrists + ankles mainly affected
Epiphyseal plates widened + irregular
Tremendous metaphysis (fraying, splaying, cupping
Spur (metaphyseal)

Wormian Bones
= intrasutural ossicles in lambdoid, posterior sagittal, temporosquamosal sutures; normal up to 6 months of age (most frequently)

Mnemonic: **"PORK CHOPS"**
  Pyknodysostosis
  Osteogenesis imperfecta
  Rickets in healing phase
  Kinky hair syndrome
  Cleidocranial dysostosis
  Hypothyroidism/Hypophosphatasia
  Otopalatodigital syndrome
  Primary acroosteolysis (Hajdu-Cheney syndrome)
  Panchydermoperiostosis/Progeria
  Syndrome of Down

Absent Greater Sphenoid Wing

Mnemonic: **"M For Marine"**
  Meningioma
  Fibrous dysplasia
  Optic glioma
  Relapsing hematoma
  Metastasis
  Aneurysm
  Retinoblastoma
  Idiopathic
  Neurofibromatosis
  Eosinophilic Granuloma

Posterior Scalloping of Vertebrae

Mnemonic: **"DAMN MALE SHAME"**
  Dermoid
  Ankylosing spondylitis
  Meningioma
  Neurofibromatosis
  Marfan syndrome
  Acromegaly
  Lipoma
  Ependymoma
  Syringohydromyelia
  Hydrocephalus
  Achondroplasia
  Mucopolysaccharidoses
  Ehlers-Danlos syndrome

INTRACRANIAL CALCIFICATIONS

Mnemonic:
  CMV calcifications are cir**cumv**entricular
  T**o**xoplasma calcifications are intrapa**r**enchymal

Calcifying Brain Tumour
Astrocytoma-calcifies less frequently but are the most
common tumor

Mnemonic: **"Ca2+ COME"**
   Craniopharyngioma
   Astrocytoma, **A**neurysm,
   Choroid plexus papilloma
   Oligodendroglioma
   Meningioma, **M**edulloblastoma
   Ependymoma

<u>Eye-of-the-Tiger Sign</u>
= markedly hypointense globus pallidus on T2W1
surrounding a higher-intensity center
   Associated with: Hallervorden-Spatz syndrome

<u>J-shaped Sella</u>

Mnemonic: **"CONMAN"**
   Chronic hydrocephalus
   Optic glioma, **O**steogenesis imperfecta
   Neurofibromatosis
   Mucopolysaccharidosis
   Achondroplasia
   Normal variant

<u>MR Appearance of Intracerebral Hematoma</u>

Mnemonic: **"DD-BD-BB-DD** ON T1/T2"

Dark-Dark	acute	0-2 days	deoxyhemoglobin
Bright-Dark	early subacute	3-7 days	intracellular methemoglobin
Bright-Bright	late subacute	8-14 days	extracellular methemoglobin
Dark-Dark	chronic	>14 days	hemosiderin

<u>LYMPHANGITIC CARCINOMATOSIS</u>

Mnemonic: **"Certain Cancers Spread By Plugging The Lymphatics"**
   Cervix
   Colon
   Stomach
   Breast
   Pancreas
   Thyroid
   Larynx

<u>Incidence of Pulmonary Metastases</u>

Mnemonic: **"CHEST"**

Choriocarcinoma	60%
Hypernephroma/Wilms tumor	30%/20%
Ewing sarcoma	18%
Sarcoma (rhabdomyo-/osteosarcoma)	21%/15%
Testicular tumor	12%

Calcifying Lung Metastases (<1%)

Mnemonic: **"BOTTOM"**
   Breast
   Osteo-/chondrosarcoma
   Thyroid (papillary)
   Testicular
   Ovarian
   Mucinous adenocarcinoma (colon)

Cavitating Lung Metastases

Mnemonic: **"Squamous Cell Metastases Tend to Cavitate"**
   Squamous cell carcinoma, **S**arcoma
   Colon
   Melanoma
   Transitional cell carcinoma
   Cervix, during **C**hemotherapy

LINITIS PLASTICA

Mnemonic: **"SLIMRAGE"**
   Scirrhous carcinoma of stomach
   Lymphoma
   Infiltration from adjacent neoplasm
   Metastasis (breast carcinoma)
   Radiation therapy
   Acids (corrosive ingestion)
   Granulomatous disease (TB, sarcoidosis, Crohn)
   Eosinophilic gastroenteritis.

Pear-shaped Urinary Bladder

Mnemonic: **"HALL"**
   Hematoma
   Aneurysm (bilateral common/external iliac artery)
   Lipomatosis
   Lymphadenopathy (pelvic)

Papillary necrosis

Mnemonic: **"POSTCARD"**
   Pyelonephritis
   Obstructive uropathy
   Sickle cell disease
   Tuberculosis, **T**rauma
   Cirrhosis = alcoholism, **C**oagulopathy
   Analgesic nephropathy
   Renal vein thrombosis
   Diabetes mellitus (50%).

<u>**Diffuse axonal injury (DAI)**</u> is a frequent result of traumatic deceleration injuries and a frequent cause of persistent vegetative state in patients. DAI is the most significant cause of morbidity in patients with traumatic brain injuries, which most commonly are the result of high-speed motor vehicle accidents. Typically, the process is diffuse and bilateral, involving the lobar white matter at the gray-white matter interface. The corpus callosum frequently is involved, as is the dorsolateral rostral brainstem. The most commonly involved area is the frontal and temporal white matter, followed by the posterior body and splenium of the corpus callosum, the caudate nuclei, thalamus, tegmentum, and internal capsule.

MRI in Meningioma

Meningiomas are usually dural-based tumors that are isoattenuating to slightly hyperattenuating. They enhance homogeneously and intensely after the injection of iodinated contrast material. Perilesional edema may be extensive. Hyperostosis and intratumoral calcifications may be present. The tumor compresses the brain without invading it. An enhancing tail involving the dura may be apparent on MRI. Meningiomas are the second most common tumor in the intradural extramedullary location, second only to tumors of the nerve sheath. Meningiomas account for approximately 25% of all spinal tumors. MRI demonstrates the intradural extramedullary location of meningiomas. Lesions are usually isointense to spinal cord on both T1-weighted and T2-weighted images. Lesions are sometimes hypointense on T1-weighted images and hyperintense on T2-weighted images.

Vein of Galen Malformation

The vein of Galen is located under the cerebral hemispheres

and drains the anterior and central regions of the brain into the sinuses of the posterior cerebral fossa. Aneurysmal malformations of the vein of Galen (VGAM) typically result in high-output congestive heart failure or may present with developmental delay, hydrocephalus, and seizures. VGAM results from an aneurysmal malformation with an arteriovenous shunting of blood. The congenital malformation develops during weeks 6-11 of fetal development as a persistent embryonic prosencephalic vein of Markowski; thus, VGAM is actually a misnomer. The vein of Markowski actually drains into the vein of Galen. VGAM usually causes high-output heart failure in the newborn resulting from the decreased resistance and high blood flow in the lesion. Associated findings include cerebral ischemic changes such as strokes or steal phenomena that result in progressive hemiparesis. Hemorrhage from the malformation can occur, although this is not a common finding. Finally, the malformation may result in mass effects, causing progressive neurological impairment. Alternatively, the malformation may cause obstruction of the cerebrospinal fluid (CSF) outflow and result in hydrocephalus.

Bohler Angle

Lateral radiographs of the foot are needed to evaluate the Bohler angle, which is the angle defined by 2 intersecting lines: one drawn from anterior process of the calcaneus to the peak of the posterior articular surface and a second drawn from the peak of the posterior articular surface to the peak of the posterior tuberosity. The average angle is 25-40°. In severe fractures with subtalar joint involvement, this angle may decrease or become negative.

Sunburst Calcification

Serous cystadenocarcinoma of pancreas.

PACS

In medical imaging, *picture archiving and communication systems (PACS)* are computers or networks dedicated to the storage, retrieval, distribution and presentation of images. The medical images are stored in an independent format. The most common format for image storage is **DICOM (Digital Imaging and Communications in Medicine)**.

SECTION SEVEN

Types of images

Most PACSs handle images from various medical imaging instruments, including ultrasound, magnetic resonance, PET, computed tomography, endoscopy, mammograms, etc

Uses

PACS replaces hard-copy based means of managing medical images, such as film archives. It expands on the possibilities of such conventional systems by providing capabilities of off-site viewing and reporting (distance education, telediagnosis). Additionally, it enables practitioners at various physical locations to access the same information simultaneously, **(teleradiology).** With the decreasing price of digital storage, PACSs provide a growing cost and space advantage over film archives. A PACS allows to store volumic exams and to reconstruct 3D images

Nephrogenic systemic fibrosis

Nephrogenic systemic fibrosis (NSF) or **Nephrogenic fibrosing dermopathy** is a rare and serious syndrome that involves fibrosis of skin, joints, eyes, and internal organs. Its cause is not fully understood, but it seems to be **associated with exposure to gadolinium** (which is frequently used as a contrast substance for MRIs) in patients with severe kidney failure. It does not have a genetic basis. In NSF, patients develop large areas of hardened skin with fibrotic nodules and plaques. Flexion contractures with an accompanying limitation of range of motion can also occur. NSF resembles scleromyxedema at the histologic (microscopic) level; it shows a proliferation of dermal fibroblasts and dendritic cells, thickened collagen bundles, increased elastic fibers, and deposits of mucin.

Most patients with NSF have undergone hemodialysis for renal failure, some have never undergone dialysis and others have received only peritoneal dialysis. Many patients have taken immunosuppressive medications and have other diseases, such as hepatitis C. Four of the five FDA-approved gadolinium contrast agents have been principally implicated in NSF, including Omniscan, Multihance, Magnevist, and OptiMARK.

The first cases of NSF were identified in 1997, but NSF was first described as an independent disease entity in 2000.

While skin involvement is on the foreground, the process may involve any organ and resembles diffuse scleroderma or systemic sclerosis. In 2006, the link between NSF and gadolinium-containing contrast agents was made. As a result, **gadolinium-containing contrast is now considered contraindicated in patients with an estimated glomerular filtration rate (a measure of renal function) under 60 and especially under 30.**

Ultrasound contrast agents

Contrast-enhanced ultrasound (CEUS) is the application of ultrasound contrast agents to traditional medical sonography. Ultrasound contrast agents are gas-filled microbubbles that are administered intravenously to the systemic circulation. Microbubbles have a high degree of echogenicity, which is the ability of an object to reflect the ultrasound waves. The echogenicity difference between the gas in the microbubbles and the soft tissue surroundings of the body is immense. Thus, ultrasonic imaging using microbubble contrast agents enhances the ultrasound backscatter, or reflection of the ultrasound waves, to produce a unique sonogram with increased contrast due to the high echogenicity difference. Contrast-enhanced ultrasound can be used to image blood perfusion in organs, measure blood flow rate in the heart and other organs, and has other applications as well.

Optison, a Food and Drug Administration (FDA)-approved microbubble made by GE Healthcare, has an albumin shell and octafluoropropane gas core. The second FDA-approved microbubble, **Levovist,** made by Schering, has a lipid/galactose shell and an air core.

Leukodystrophy refers to a group of disorders characterized by progressive degeneration of the white matter of the brain. The leukodystrophies are caused by imperfect growth or development of the myelin sheath, the fatty covering that acts as an insulator around nerve fibers. Myelin, which the white matter of the brain takes its colour from, is a complex substance made up of at least ten different chemicals. Each of the leukodystrophies is the result of a defect in the gene that controls the production or metabolism of one (and only one) of the component molecules of myelin.

Specific leukodystrophies include.

- **Adrenoleukodystrophy-** (also known as Addison-Schilder Disease or Sudanophilic Leukodystrophy) is a rare, inherited disorder that leads to progressive brain damage, failure of the adrenal glands and eventually death.

- **Metachromatic leukodystrophy-**Metachromatic leukodystrophy (MLD, also called Arylsulfatase A deficiency) is the most common form of a family of genetic diseases known as the leukodystrophies, diseases which affect the growth

- **Krabbe disease-**also known as globoid cell leukodystrophy or galactosylceramide lipidosis. Subcortical U fibers are spared. Thalami show altered signal.

- **Canavan disease-** Macrocephaly, Canavan disease is caused by a defective *ASPA* gene which is responsible for the production of the enzyme aspartoacylase This enzyme breaks down the concentrated brain molecule *N*-acetyl aspartate.

- **Alexander disease-** Macrocephaly, involvment of white matter with frontal lobe predominance

MR spectroscopy

MR spectroscopy is a noninvasive means of obtaining metabolic information. MRI is a technique used for the noninvasive detection and anatomical mapping of water protons (hydrogen), whereas MR spectroscopy records protons in intrinsic phosphorus-containing metabolites, sodium, potassium, carbon, nitrogen, and fluorine.

Metabolites

The most prominent resonance in a proton spectrum is NAA. The presence of NAA is attributable to its N-acetyl methyl group, which resonates at 2 ppm. **NAA is accepted as a neuronal marker; as such, its concentration will decrease with many insults to the brain (such as neoplasms, infarcts, epilepsy, and dementia. There is a marked increase in NAA peaks in Canavan diseases**

Creatine resonates at 3.03 ppm and contains contributions from creatine, creatine phosphate, and, to a lesser degree, gaminobutyric acid, lysine, and glutathione. An additional peak for creatine may be visible at 3.94 ppm. **Therefore, the creatine peak is sometimes referred to as total creatine; it represents the energy source.**

The peak for choline occurs at 3.2 ppm. These compounds are involved in the synthesis and degradation of cell membranes, and their concentration may be affected in disorders that influence membrane turnover. **Therefore, increased choline probably reflects increased membrane synthesis and/or an increased number of cells, as seen in tumors.**

Percutaneous Vertebroplasty: New Treatment for Vertebral Compression Fractures

Percutaneous vertebroplasty is a newer technique in which acrylic cement is injected through a needle into a collapsed or weakened vertebra to stabilize the fracture. This procedure is effective for treating certain types of painful vertebral compression fractures and some painful or unstable benign and malignant vertebral lesions that fail to respond to the traditional conservative therapies. Most experts believe that pain relief is achieved through mechanical support and stability provided by the bone cement. The semisolid mixture of polymethylmethacrylate (PMMA), an acrylic cement used in orthopedic procedures, has been shown **to restore strength and stiffness in vertebral bodies in postmortem studies**

MDCT angiography in Pulmonary embolism

Computed tomography with radiocontrast, effectively a pulmonary angiogram imaged by CT and also known as CT pulmonary angiography (CTPA), is increasingly used as the mainstay in diagnosis. Assessing the accuracy of CT pulmonary angiography is hindered by the rapid changes in the number of rows of detectors available in multidetector CT (MDCT) machines. A study with a mixture of 4 slice and 16 slice scanners reported a sensitivity of 83% and a specificity of 96%. This study noted that additional testing is necessary when the clinical probability is inconsistent with the imaging results. MDCT has progressed to be available with 64 slices, each 0.625 mm thick. These machines take 3-4 seconds to scan and may be gated to the heart beat. The sensitivity and specificity of these machines are much better.

SECTION SEVEN

Recent recommendations for a diagnostic algorithm have been published by the PIOPED investigators;

- Low clinical probability. If negative D-dimer, PE is excluded. If positive D-dimer, obtain MDCT and based treatment on results.

- Moderate clinical probability. If negative D-dimer, PE is excluded. *However*, the authors were not concerned that a negative MDCT with negative D-dimer in this setting has an 5% probability of being false. Presumably, the 5% error rate will fall as 64 slice MDCT is more commonly used. If positive D-dimer, obtain MDCT and based treatment on results.

- **High clinical probability. Proceed to MDCT. If positive, treat, if negative, addition tests are needed to exclude PE.**

Doppler in IUGR

Doppler evaluation has a role in high risk pregnancies with parameters reflecting the placental resistance and blood flow. Umbilical artery is a low resistance vessel which has forward flow in both systole and diastole. However, in IUGR the diastolic flow reduces and S/D ratio is increased. Absence of end-diastolic flow or reversal of flow are indications for termination. Changes in the flow velocity waveforms of umbilical artery are important in the management of high risk pregnancies. Other vessels which are studied are uterine artery and Fetal MCA. Persistence of diastolic notch beyond 24-26 weeks of POG is a marker for high risk pregnancy particularly in cases of PIH

Hybrid Imaging

The clinical use of positron emission tomographic/computed tomographic (PET/CT) and single photon emission computed tomographic (SPECT)/CT hybrid imaging systems is expected to increase dramatically in the near future. **Thus they provide both functional and anatomical information.**

Positron emission tomography (PET) is a nuclear medicine imaging technique which produces a three-dimensional image or map of functional processes in the body. The system detects pairs of gamma rays emitted indirectly by a positron-emitting radionuclide (tracer), which is introduced into the body on a biologically active molecule. PET scans are increasingly read alongside CT the combination (**"co-registration"**) giving both anatomic and metabolic. Radionuclides used in PET scanning are typically isotopes with short half lives such as carbon-11 (~20 min), nitrogen-13 (~10 min), oxygen-15 (~2 min), and fluorine-18 (~110 min). These radionuclides are incorporated either into compounds normally used by the body such as glucose (or glucose analogues), water or ammonia, or into molecules that bind to receptors or other sites of drug action. Limitations to the widespread use of PET arise from the high costs of **cyclotrons needed to produce the short-lived radionuclides** for PET scanning and the need for specially adapted on-site chemical synthesis apparatus to produce the radiopharmaceuticals. FDG-PET can be used for diagnosis, staging, and monitoring treatment of cancers, **particularly in Hodgkin's disease, non Hodgkin's lymphoma, and lung cancer. Rubidium-82, which can be created in a portable generator and is used for myocardial perfusion studies.**

PET scanning is non-invasive, but it does involve exposure to ionizing radiation. The total dose of radiation is small, however, usually around 7 mSv.

Aberrant subclavian artery

Anomalous origin from the proximal descending aorta of either the right or left subclavian artery. An aberrant right subclavian artery arises distal to the left aortic arch. An aberrant left subclavian artery arises distal to the right aortic arch (non-mirror-image right aortic arch); an aortic diverticulum exists at the site of origin. In a right arch with aberrant left subclavian artery, a right-sided ligamentum arteriosum connects the diverticulum and the proximal left pulmonary artery producing a complete vascular ring. In both types of aberrant subclavian arteries, the vessel runs behind the oesophagus. The aberrant right subclavian artery produces an impression on the back of the oesophagus while the left one usually causes anterior displacement and severe compression of the oesophagus. The latter also frequently causes airway compression. The right aberrant artery can be associated with dysphagia in adults while the left usually causes symptomatic airway and oesophageal obstruction during infancy or early childhood.

SECTION SEVEN

Plain radiography with barium swallow displays a right-sided aortic arch impression and posterior impression of the aberrant left subclavian on the oesophagus or left-sided aortic arch impression and posterior impression of the aberrant left subclavian artery on the oesophagus. The lateral view also reveals anterior displacement and compression of the trachea by the aberrant left subclavian artery. Thoracic aortography demonstrates the relationship of the arch to the trachea or oesophagus (simultaneous barium swallow) and origin of the aberrant subclavian as the fourth major branch of the aortic arch.

Radiology for vascular rings

Patients, especially infants or young children, with recurrent respiratory symptoms such as chronic cough, stridor and wheeze, should be examined for the possible presence of congenital vascular rings. Contrast-enhanced CT can clearly show the anatomy of vascular rings. Contrast-enhanced thoracic ct with 3d reconstruction may allow accurate diagnosis and clearly show compression of the tracheoesophageal tract. For several decades, the diagnosis of vascular rings has mainly relied on chest X-rays and barium swallow. Recently, it has been shown that CT had replaced barium swallow as the diagnostic procedure of choice for vascular ring evaluation. Although angiography has been used to further delineate arch anatomy, it is now rarely performed due to the availability of noninvasive techniques and due to problems like overlapping of structures.

Delta sign

Empty delta sign is seen in a patient with superior sagittal sinus thrombosis. Transverse contrast-enhanced CT image reveals low-attenuating thrombus within the superior sagittal sinus, surrounded by a triangular area of enhancement.

Tear drop sign

The floor of the orbit is the most common portion of the orbit to sustain fracture. A classic radiographic finding in blow-out fractures is the presence of a polypoid mass (the tear-drop) protruding from the floor of the orbit into the maxillary antrum the tear-drop represents the herniated orbital contents, periorbital fat and inferior rectus muscle.

Section 8

Appendices

APPENDIX A

ISOTOPES USED IN MEDICINE

Reactor Radioisotopes

Molybdenum-99 (66 h): Used as the 'parent' in a generator to produce technetium-99m.

Technetium-99m (6 h): Used in to image the skeleton and heart muscle in particular, but also for brain, thyroid, lungs (perfusion and ventilation), liver, spleen, kidney (structure and filtration rate), gall bladder, bone marrow, salivary and lacrimal glands, heart blood pool, infection and numerous specialised medical studies.

Bismuth-213 (46 min): Used for TAT.

Chromium-51 (28 d): Used to label red blood cells and quantify gastro-intestinal protein loss.

Cobalt-60 (10.5 mth): Formerly used for external beam radiotherapy.

Copper-64 (13 h): Used to study genetic diseases affecting copper metabolism, such as Wilson's and Menke's diseases.

Dysprosium-165 (2 h): Used as an aggregated hydroxide for synovectomy treatment of arthritis.

Erbium-169 (9.4 d): Use for relieving arthritis pain in synovial joints.

Holmium-166 (26 h): Being developed for diagnosis and treatment of liver tumours.

Iodine-125 (60 d): Used in cancer brachytherapy (prostate and brain), also diagnostically to evaluate the filtration rate of kidneys and to diagnose deep vein thrombosis in the leg. It is also widely used in radioimmuno-assays to show the presence of hormones in tiny quantities.

Iodine-131 (8 d): Widely used in treating thyroid cancer and in imaging the thyroid; also in diagnosis of abnormal liver function, renal (kidney) blood flow and urinary tract obstruction. A strong gamma emitter, but used for beta therapy.

Iridium-192 (74 d): Supplied in wire form for use as an internal radiotherapy source for cancer treatment (used then removed).

Iron-59 (46 d): Used in studies of iron metabolism in the spleen.

Lutetium-177 (6.7 d): Lu-177 is increasingly important as it emits just enough gamma for imaging while the beta radiation does the therapy on small (eg endocrine) tumours. Its half-life is long enough to allow sophisticated preparation for use.

Palladium-103 (17 d): Used to make brachytherapy permanent implant seeds for early stage prostate cancer.

Phosphorus-32 (14 d): Used in the treatment of polycythemia vera (excess red blood cells). Beta emitter.

Potassium-42 (12 h): Used for the determination of exchangeable potassium in coronary blood flow.

Rhenium-186 (3.8 d): Used for pain relief in bone cancer. Beta emitter with weak gamma for imaging.

Rhenium-188 (17 h): Used to beta irradiate coronary arteries from an angioplasty balloon.

Samarium-153 (47 h): Sm-153 is very effective in relieving the pain of secondary cancers lodged in the bone, sold as Quadramet. Also very effective for prostate and breast cancer. Beta emitter.

Selenium-75 (120 d): Used in the form of seleno-methionine to study the production of digestive enzymes.

Sodium-24 (15 h): For studies of electrolytes within the body.

Strontium-89 (50 d): Very effective in reducing the pain of prostate and bone cancer. Beta emitter.

Xenon-133 (5 d): Used for pulmonary (lung) ventilation studies.

Ytterbium-169 (32 d): Used for cerebrospinal fluid studies in the brain.

Ytterbium-177 (1.9 h): Progenitor of Lu-177.

Yttrium-90 (64 h): Used for cancer brachytherapy and as silicate colloid for the relieving the pain of arthritis in larger synovial joints. Pure beta emitter.

Radioisotopes of caesium, gold and ruthenium are also used in brachytherapy

Cyclotron Radioisotopes

Carbon-11, Nitrogen-13, Oxygen-15, Fluorine-18: These are positron emitters used in PET for studying brain physiology and pathology, in particular for localising epileptic focus, and in dementia, psychiatry and neuropharmacology studies. They also have a significant role in cardiology. F-18 in FDG has become very important in detection of cancers and the monitoring of progress in their treatment, using PET.

Cobalt-57 (272 d): Used as a marker to estimate organ size and for in-vitro diagnostic kits.

Gallium-67 (78 h): Used for tumour imaging and localisation of inflammatory lesions (infections).

Indium-111 (2.8 d): Used for specialist diagnostic studies, eg brain studies, infection and colon transit studies.

Iodine-123 (13 h): Increasingly used for diagnosis of thyroid function, it is a gamma emitter without the beta radiation of I-131.

Krypton-81m (13 sec) from Rubidium-81 (4.6 h): Kr-81m gas can yield functional images of pulmonary ventilation, e.g. in asthmatic patients, and for the early diagnosis of lung diseases and function.

Rubidium-82 (65 h): Convenient PET agent in myocardial perfusion imaging.

Strontium-92 (25 d): Used as the 'parent' in a generator to produce Rb-82.

Thallium-201 (73 h): Used for diagnosis of coronary artery disease other heart conditions such as heart muscle death and for location of low-grade lymphomas.

APPENDIX B

Radiopharmaceuticals currently used and their
common clinical applications

Organ system	Clinical application	Radiopharma-ceutical	Biological behaviour
Cardio-vascular system Myocardial perfusion	Detection of ischaemia, infarction, and viability assessment	^{201}Tl (thallous) chloride)	K+ analogue extracted in proportion to bloodflow
		^{99m}Tc isonitriles	Cationic complexes taken up by myocytes in proportion to blood flow
		^{99m}Tc teboroxime	Lipophilic compound which accumulates by diffusion
		^{99m}Tc phosphines	Uptake propor-tional to blood flow
Myocardial metabolism	Viability assessment	^{123}I fatty acids	Enters primary metabolic path-way in viable cells: limited catabolism
		^{18}F-deoxyglucose	Enter metabolic pathway in viable cells demonstra-tes secondary shift to anaerobic glycolysis
Cardiac ventriculo-graphy	Quantifica-tion of right and left ventricular function at rest and with exercise Detection of wall motion abnormalities	^{99m}Tc-red blood cells	Characteriza-tion of cardiac chambers motion, locali-zation of red cells within cardiac chambers
		^{99m}Tc-albumin	

Contd.

Contd.

	Quantification and detection of shunts (and valvar regurgitation)		
Cellular blood components			
Red blood cells	Detection of haemangioma	99m Tc-labelled red blood cells	Red cell pooling
	Cardiac ventriculography Gastrointestinal bleeding Red cell survival	51 Cr (Sodium chromate)	Red cell extravasation Red cell disappearance form the blood
White blood cells	Localization of sites of infection or inflammation	99m Tc-111 In-labelled cells 99m Tc-labelled antigranulocyte antibody	Cellular diapedesis
Platelets	Platelet survival Localization of sites of active thrombosis	111 In-labelled platelets	Platelet sequestration and degradation
Central nervous system			
Cerebral blood flow	Blood flow distribution	99m Tc-HMPAO	Diffusion through the blood–brain barrier (BBB) and brain extraction
	tumours? seizure disorders? dementia? brain death studies?	99m Tc-ECD	
	Regional blood flow at rest and upon activation	H_2 ^{15} O	BBB diffusible flow tracer

Contd.

SECTION EIGHT

Contd.

Cerebral metabolism	Functional and regional mapping of neuronal activity at rest at rest? upon activation? during seizure? in the interictal state?	[18] F-deoxyglucose	Enter metabolic pathway in viable cells
	Staging of brain tumour	[18] F-deoxyglucose	
	Follow-up of therapy	[201] TI	
Cerebrospinal fluid	CSF shunt patency	[111] In-DTPA	Follows cerebral spinal fluid (CSF) flow dynamics
	Localization of CSF leaks Differentiation of normal pressure hydrocephaly from atrophy		

Gastrointestinal system

Liver-spleen imaging	Space-occupying lesions, organ sizing, RES function	[99m] Tc-sulphur colloid	Phagocytosis by reticulo-endothelial cells
Spleen imaging	Detection of ectopic splenic tissue	Heat-damaged [99m] Tc-labelled red blood cells	Splenic trapping of damaged cells
Hepatobiliary imaging	Assessment of biliary ducts patency	[99m] Tc-iminodiacetic acid derivatives	Active uptake—follows bilirubin conjugation and excretion pathway
	Evaluation of gallbladder contractility Diagnosis of acute vs chronic cholecystitis		

Contd.

Contd.

	Differentiation between biliary atresia and neonatal hepatitis		
Bowel transit studies	Oesophageal transit and reflux	^{99m} Tc-sulphur colloid	Transit of labelled material
	Gastric emptying and antral motility	^{99m} Tc-sulphur colloid	Compartmental localization of labelled material
	Gastric emptying	^{111} In-DTPA $^{13 \text{ or } 14}$ C-labelled substrates	Detection in breath of exhaled $^{13 \text{ or } 14}$ CO_2 metabolite
	Duodeno-gastric reflux	^{99m} Tc-imino-diacetic acid derivatives	Bile detection and localization
	Small bowel and colon transit	^{111} In-DTPA	Transit of labelled material
		$^{13 \text{ or } 14}$ C-labelled substrates	Detection in breath of exhaled $^{13 \text{ or } 14}$ CO_2 metabolite
Helicobacter pylori (HP) infection	Detection of HP urease production	$^{13 \text{ or } 14}$ C-labelled urea	Detection in breath of exhaled $^{13 \text{ or } 14}$ CO_2 metabolite
Gastro-intestinal bleeding	Acute and chronic bleeding	^{99m} Tc-sulphur colloid	Extravasation in the bowel
		^{99m} Tc-labelled red cells	
Perito-neovenous shunts	Determination of shunt patency	^{99m} Tc-sulphur colloid	Compartmental localization
Salivary glands	Evaluation of salivary function and ducts patency	^{99m} Tc-pertechnetate	Active uptake and secretion

Contd.

SECTION EIGHT

Contd.

Gastric mucosa	Detection and localization of a Meckel's diverticulum containing gastric mucosa	^{99m} Tc-pertechnetate	Active uptake by gastric mucosa
Genitourinary system			
Renal perfusion	Evaluation of arterial blood flow Diagnosis of transplant rejection	^{99m} Tc-DTPA ^{99m} Tc-MAG3 ^{99m} Tc-DTPA	Early intra-vascular localization
Renal function	GFR measurement Measure-ment of effective renal plasma flow; tubular function	^{51} Cr-EDTA ^{99m} Tc-MAG3	Clearance by glomerular filtration Tubular uptake
Renal mor-phology	Detection of renal infarct Global renal morphology	^{99m} Tc-DMSA	Retention in renal cortex
Bladder	Quantitation of bladder residual vesicoureteral reflux	^{99m} Tc-DTPA	Compartmental localization
Scrotum	Differentia-tion between acute testicular torsion and epididymitis	^{99m} Tc-pertechnate	Early intra-vascular localization
Pulmonary system			
Ventilation scan	Evaluation of regional ventilation	^{133} Xe gas ^{81} Kr^m gas ^{99m} Tc aérosols	Distributes in lungs in propor-tion to regional ventilation

Contd.

Contd.

Perfusion scan	Detection of pulmonary emboli, right to left shunts; preoperative and transplant evaluation of relative lung perfusion	^{99m} Tc albumin macroaggregates	Pulmonary capillary blockade
Paren-chymal tissue	Interstitial lung disease staging and therapeutic evaluation	^{67} Ga	Binds to transferrin in the intravascular compartment, taken up by cells of the inflamma-tory response, binds to lacto-ferrin andferritin and concentrates in lysosomes
Musculo-skeletal system	Detection of soft tissue vs primary bone disorders during Phases I and II of study	^{99m} Tc-poly-phosphate compounds	Intravascular and early soft tissue distribution (Phase I and II)
	Detection of benign, malignant, and infectious bone lesions		Fixed to hydro-xyapatite crystals (Phase III)

Thyroid-parathyroid

Thyroid	Evaluation of gland size, morphology and function (uptake).	Iodine-123	Active uptake (^{123} I and ^{99m} Tc) followed by organification (^{123} I)
		^{99m} Tc-perte-chnetate	
	Determination of functional status of nodules		
	Detection of thyroid cancer and	Iodine-131	Active uptake and organification

Contd.

Contd.

	metastases, thyroid cancer treatment		
Parathyroid	Localization of parathyroid adenoma and carcinoma	^{99m} Tc-MIBI	Cationic complexes taken up in proportion to blood flow and trapped in mitochondria

Tumour markers

Neuro-endocrine tissue	Somatostatin receptor positive tumours	^{111} In-pentetreotide (Octecotide®)	Binds to somatostatin receptors
Lympho-poietic tissue	Staging and localization of lymphoma	^{67} Ga (gallium citrate)	Binds to transferrin in the intra-vascular compartment, taken up by cancer cells, binds to lactoferrin and ferritin, and concentrates in lysosomes
Brain neoplasia chloride)	Brain tumour staging and therapeutic follow up	^{201} Tl (thallous chloride)	Concentrates in tumour cells following BBB damage
Adeno-carcinoma	Tumour detection and staging	^{111} In-Satumomab pendetide	Antigen-antibody recognition
Miscellaneous neoplasia	Tumour detection and staging	^{18} F-deoxyglucose	Uptake proportional to tumour glucose metabolism

Opinions of a few PG aspirants...

1. Good things come in small packages. *Review of Radiology* is a book that lives up to this adage and more... This book has the unique quality of being all inclusive, yet in a manner that allows efficient utilization of time...Within a few hours, it gives you a feeling of one subject under your belt... Kudos to the author for aiding overburdened students to scale one hurdle with relative ease...

2. Hats off to book on radiology–very comprehensive, authentic and manageable in small time. The information is very comprehensive and very high yielding...

3. The success of the author lies in the fact that he has been able to give SO MUCH OF THE "NEEDED" POINTS in so few pages...Most of the points that are given in the book have been already asked and more importantly almost all questions that have been previously asked can be solved with this little book... This book is bound to be one of the classics of PG Preparatory... "This book can be read at the cost and time of two movies" and to answer 100% in State PG and about 90% (87.5% to me more accurate) in All India (where you are expected to answer 66% correctly to get into the top 100 ranks) from such a small book is commendable and the author needs to be appreciated.

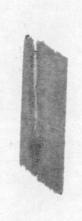